KAVA

Nature's Relaxant
For Anxiety, Stress and Pain

Hasnain Walji, Ph.D.

Hohm Press
Prescott, Arizona

Cover design: Kim Johansen
Layout and design: Visual Perspectives, Phoenix, AZ

ISBN: 0-934252-78-5

Library of Congress Catalogue Card Number: 97-077115

Hohm Press
P.O. Box 2501
Prescott, AZ 86302
800-381-2700
http://www.booknotes.com/hohm/

Contents

The Shifting Paradigm

The dominant medical system in the West (allopathic medicine) attempts to cure disease once it has become established, in other words: the illness approach. A single treatment, or protocol (typically a medicinal formula, "a pill for every ill") is matched with the disease, often regardless of the uniqueness of the patient who has the disease.

In contrast, we have the holistic model. In this wellness approach the physician and/or patient primarily seeks to maintain the state of health (*homeostasis*) and, thereby, prevent disease by denying it the opportunity to take hold. Or, if disease has already taken hold, the physician or patient attempts to lend additional support to the natural or innate healing system of the body.

Wellness includes positive steps towards taking responsibility for our own personal well-being. We know ourselves better than anyone else possibly can.

It is no longer expedient to remain passive about taking care of ourselves, expecting a "quick fix." The myth of "a pill for every ill" should be abandoned, whether the pill is composed of synthetic ingredients, inert materials or wild-crafted herbs. The wellness movement is not just about replacing drugs with herbs.

In 1993 a landmark study appeared in the prestigious *New England Journal of Medicine*. The lead author, Dr. David Eisenberg, a Harvard-based physician who had enjoyed an eye-opening medical education in China, revealed for the first time just how extensive the "alternative underground" had become. One out of every three U.S. citizens was a consumer of alternative products or methodologies, involving more than thirteen billion dollars. Indeed, patient visits to alternative practitioners exceeded visits to primary care physicians. The most recent estimate is even higher— a 50:50 split. Today the average U.S. citizen is as likely as not to use alternative medicine.

The Eisenberg study may have been more of an indicator of the therapies of the future than we initially discerned. Exercise (26%) and prayer (25%) were utilized the most, while megavitamin therapy (2%) and herbs (3%) were insignificant. This is as it should be! Holistic healing is all about potentiating our inner healing powers (prayers and meditation do this, for example), rather than by using outside interventions even if they be natural remedies. The Eisenberg study seems to point towards that end. It seems that our future health lies not with increased technology, including refined transplant techniques, additional organs (from pigs, or clones etc.), more powerful drugs (to overcome rejection), or even with finding the funds to pay for every eligible person. Rather, our future lies in lowering the demand for intervention, notably through the reduction of self-abuse. Happily, the paradigm shift to wellness has begun. This book in common with the twenty others that I have written is part of that shift.

It is abundantly clear that people cannot be well if they are inactive, nor if they are spiritually unsatisfied. Does this mean that personal trainers and priests should be covered by health insurance? (It would probably be a sound investment!) Realistically, if people are well, their work will be more productive and, hopefully, rewarding. This, combined with lower expenditures on illness, should provide each of us with more discretionary income to cover wellness "luxuries" like herbs, vitamins and manual therapies.

However, there are some inherently sinister aspects of the transition from the illness approach to the new paradigm of wellness medicine. Notably the attempt to transform herbs into "phytopharmaceuticals" manufactured by the pharmaceutical industry and available only by prescription. This would preserve the status quo of the pharmaceutical industry and the role of physicians as its "gatekeepers." Typical arguments supporting this view include:

- the need to control the processing of herbs in order to obtain a standardized extract;

- the need to protect the public from dangerous herbs or potent extracts;
- the need to protect the public from erroneous diagnoses;
- the need to protect the public from exploitation;

Fortunately, the U.S. population is still considered to be capable of deciding how to spend some of its own health dollars. This was partly by default. It was probably assumed that low cost, out-of-pocket health care did not comprise a significant proportion of health expenditure and could be safely ignored. In short, there was no money in it!

A more palatable "spin" for public consumption revolves around the stereotype of "alternative" health-care as being essentially worthless and only practiced by "quacks" or charlatans. Only unlicensed health providers, "maverick" physicians or "medical heretics" would pursue such avenues. Surely, no self-respecting licensed physician would indulge in such practices, at any price.

Kava use should not be thought of as a panacea for all ills, nor as a magic pill. In this book I have tried to look at the use of this herb from a holistic perspective.

Did You Know?

CHAPTER ONE

Introduction

Kava is a fairly new item on the shelves of health stores. So new, in fact, you still might not know anything about it; at least from the name. Anyone who has taken an interest in the cultures of the South Pacific may have a vague recollection (from old newsreels, for example, which accompanied movies at one time) of a ceremonial drink offered to honored guests, like the Queen of England or President Lyndon Johnson. For most of us, it would be one time we wouldn't want to change places with these dignitaries! The commentary would go something like this:

The Queen arrives in Fiji aboard the royal yacht Britannia *and is greeted by a ceremony in which she must down the first cup of the local beverage. Villagers traditionally prepared the drink for several days, chewing leaves of a local bush and spitting the residue into a bucket to allow it to ferment....*

Only those with a firm constitution could bear to watch the Queen fulfill her obligations, for which she would be (deservedly) applauded by the villagers.

In fact, this ceremonial beverage, throughout Oceania, is the main use for kava, or kava-kava, in one form or another, depending upon which island the ceremony took place. In Hawaii it was known as *awa*. In Fiji the term is *yaqona* (pronounced yangona). (See separate section on etymology later in this chapter.) Of course, the preparations on the shelf at your local store are not prepared in the traditional way! Nor do they take this traditional form. We are more likely to consume a pill—which protects us from the strange taste and effects of kava (like many other medicines)—than to develop a taste for it. Certainly, it is much easier for most of us in the West to import an herb, without the total cultural experience. Briefly, a Westernized relationship to kava may be likened to our relationship to drinking tea. In many Western countries people commonly drink tea, hot or iced, just as they would any other beverage. In Japan, however, the small cup of green tea is much more potent and is surrounded by a great deal of ceremonial.

Stories about the making and drinking of kava were first brought back to Europe following voyages of exploration, notably those of Captain James Cook during the mid-eighteenth century, although the true origins have been lost in antiquity. In some cultures throughout the Pacific the practice of kava usage was virtually eradicated during the nineteenth century by the influx of Christian missionaries, which followed rapidly upon the exploration. The inhabitants of many islands have resumed the practice quite recently, spurred on as well to develop kava as a major cash crop for export, notably to Germany, which takes fifty tons annually, largely to become a standardized herbal extract.

Sales of the extract within Germany, alone, now reach eight million dollars annually. To place this in perspective, while it is a considerable sum, especially to the native producer in Vanuatu [an island country of the southern Pacific Ocean east of northern Australia], the number-one product, four-fold ahead of its nearest competitor, is Ginkgo biloba ($284 million).

Essentially, therefore, kava is an exotic drink surviving from the distant past, but it is now also established as a plant- (or "phyto"-) medicine, replete with all the chemical analyses and double-blind, randomized controlled trials of modern Western medical science.

But, let's not get ahead of ourselves! Probably the first thing should be to identify the kava plant.

Botanical Characteristics

Kava (or *Piper methisticum*), whether it is used for a beverage or medicine, is derived from the plant species with the same name (*see also* Etymology) belonging to the pepper family (*Piperaceae*). The active ingredients are concentrated within its roots, which, when consumed in liberal amounts, produce a state of drunkenness (hence: *methisticum*).

The formal botanical name was conferred by G. Forster (the botanist aboard Cook's second voyage) and is simply the Latin form of "intoxicating pepper." The botanical citation is properly written as P. methysticum G. Forst.

Kava requires a warm, moist climate and forms dense thickets, six feet high (or more, up to twenty feet in ideal conditions). Its large green leaves are somewhat heart shaped, resembling also those of a pond lily, six to eight inches in length. Mature plants may be 3 - 5 years old, although most commercial crops use the faster maturing varieties (2½ - 3 years). Maturation seems to affect the strength and flavor of the product obtained from the root.

Plants do have male and female flowers, although these are sterile, so plants are propagated vegetatively, either by dividing the roots, or, like sugar cane, by planting a section of the stalk. First small sections of stalks are placed within a heavily watered trench (a mud hole) until they sprout. Once sprouted they are transferred into the ground. This means that the plant must be cultivated by human labor and is a human creation. Kava may have been domesticated and cultivated for over two thousand years.

In creating the preparation, the whole plant is dug up and the tops removed, leaving only the roots which may extend two or more feet in depth. The root system is a knotted mass weighing as much as one hundred pounds, while individual roots may be as wide as your hand (5 - 8 cms / 2 - 4 inches). (Preparation of the root is considered separately, later.)

Each island cultivating kava will have a stock of tens of thousands of mature trees. Maturity for domestic use tends to be around seven years, minimum; while kava marked for export will be considered "mature" earlier. After all, exported kava will usually not be judged on its flavor, like grapeseed processed for nutritional purposes as distinct from wine for connoisseurs, or instant coffee compared to one's favorite "java."

According to Vincent Lebot (a French geneticist and tropical plant breeder who has authored a number of books and articles on the subject), kava may be a cultivated derivative from *Piper wichmanni*, which is also indigenous to Vanuatu.

A number of different varieties of kava have been identified, up to seventy-two in Vanuatu (formerly New Hebrides, northeast of Australia) alone. Differentiation is made by the green of the leaves, or the color of the stalks: including spotted, white, red and green. Differences have been substantiated by chemical analysis. A small green variety from Western New Guinea, for example, reputed to be more potent than a larger red variety, did, indeed, contain more dihydrokawain. (Chemistry is considered separately.)

Origins

Anthropologists have been debating the origins of both the people of Polynesia and their plants since Cook's voyages brought them to the notice of Western academia. The debate is no closer to closure now than at any time in the past. Within the field of anthropology, the term "ethnobotany" would be more specific to this particular field, bringing together, as it does, the people *and* their plants.

Certainly, within Oceania, there are cultural similarities to the dominant cultures of India and China, including the ritualistic drinking of soma and tea, respectively. However the kava plant itself, seems to have originated, either in some of the Pacific islands, or no further west than Indonesia.

New Guinea is another favorite area for kava growth. It is the largest remaining land mass in the region and provides both major forms of plant stimulants: kava and betel.

Betel is a rather more potent and complex habit than kava. Even in some areas where it is available, the local population has, curiously, not taken up the habit. One reason may be that it requires three different ingredients: the crushed nut (actually the seed) from the betel palm (Areca catechu) and leaves of another pepper tree (*Piper betle*) taken with slaked lime. It is also held in the mouth, rather like chewing tobacco, where it turns the mouth blood red (reacting with the saliva), as well as stains the teeth. Whether the

Samoans do not care for the laborious process of assembling the different ingredients, or the side-effects, or simply do not need the additional stimulation, is difficult to say. There may be a local taboo (*tabu*) against it, or an origin story, which encouraged the use of betel, may be lacking.

The origin stories for kava are most intriguing, for our purposes.

Origin Stories

Traditional people around the world may have lacked an alphabet or written language, but they have a rich supply of stories which have been passed down through the millennia. Some myths from diverse cultures are interestingly similar. For example, the people of Oceania share aspects of a myth with Native Americans, referring to the same group of stars, known to us as the Pleiades. We could also, by "*stretching* a point," say that the Pentecost islanders have bungee-jumping in common with more adventurous Westerners! (The islanders leap from platforms with vines around their ankles to commemorate an ancient legend.)

A well-known authority on kava, Dr. Yadhu Singh, who grew up in Fiji and is now a professor of pharmacy at South Dakota State University, has related several legends in his publications.

Each culture has its own version of an origin story making claim to kava. One legend has it that the kava root first grew from the grave of a Tongan leper. There is some substance to this, in that an over-indulgence in kava, to the deficit of good nutrition, will result in a skin disease. Ancient wisdom may, simply, be reinforcing the virtues of good nutrition and sobriety. At one time kava was reserved for special occasions—a message for "moderation in all things."

In this Tongan legend, the great chief Loau visited his servant Feva'anga. The servant wished to honor his chief with a feast, but had nothing to give, except his daughter, Kava'onau, who suffered from leprosy. Chief Loau refused to partake of the meal, however, and gave instructions that the food should be placed in the ground and used to prepare a drink. That ceremony, associated with kava, therefore, may be compared, in Western tradition, with taking communion. Kava has been the lifeblood of these societies.

Dr. Scott Norton, a dermatologist based in Honolulu, provides us with a version in the melodic, Tongan language, so we may enjoy the "ring" of authenticity:

Pea koia 'oku inu ai ae kava o lahi pea fisi o hange ha kilia, he koe tupu ae kava mei he fefine na'e kilia.
[And those that drink much kava become scaly, like a leper, just as the kava grew from the body of a leprous woman.]

Actually, "Pidgin English"—the English slang from the sailors—still dominates many cultures in the Pacific region, and can be found on the sign board outside a kava drinking establishment (nakamal). Kava, on these signs, may be referred to as "grog," like the rum of the Navy, while the owner of the kava-drinking establishment may declare to passersby that he hopes to: *"Welkam yu long eni taem nouo!"* (Welcome you along any time now!) And promises that his beverage will help provide drinkers with: "Long laef blong yu." [A long life belongs to you.]

Several other tales link kava drinking with chiefs, or even gods. In a Samoan tale (the society made famous by the work of anthropologist, Margaret Mead) the god, Tangaloa, came down to earth and wanted some kava to drink. He sent his assistants back to heaven for some of the root. They mistakenly brought back the whole plant. Tangaloa took his root and discarded the rest, which grew luxuriantly.

The Samoans also have an explanation for how they obtained kava (and sugar cane) from the Fijians. A girl went to Fiji as the bride of a great chief. As she prepared to visit her homeland she climbed a hill and pondered what gifts to take with her. She noticed a rat chewing one plant (sugar cane) and seeming to be lulled into a sleep. "This plant must be very comforting," she thought, "my people will enjoy this gift."

When the rat awoke, it went straight for a nearby plant (kava). It became more lively. The two plants complimented one another perfectly, so she realized that she should take them both back to Samoa. The Samoans took readily to their new plants and were able to disperse them further afield, swapping some for hens. The Samoans, then, were probably the first to recognize the value of these plants. They propagated kava and shared kava plants with the other islands, which contributed enormously to the economy of their whole region.

The Polynesians made incredible journeys up, down and across the Pacific, so they may very well have simply carried the kava plant stock with them wherever they settled. After all, adult men the world over seem to have a taste for something other than water, or coconut milk, however delicious and beneficial such substances may be in a virgin world.

Etymology

Kava kava (*kava* for short) is the Polynesian term for the plant (Piper methysticum), the beverage derived from it and the ceremonies associated with it. Brunton (1989) informs us that ethnographers have traced kava through hundreds of Melanesian languages to a proto-Oceanic name: *kawa*. Several languages possess terms that are quite obviously related, such as *'awa* (in Hawaii), while others are more distant etymologically: *yaqona* (Samoan), or *seka* in Kosrae, or *sakau* (Pohnpei or Ponape), *gea* in the Bank islands, and *gi* in the Torres Islands. Each dialect, of which there are several dozen, seems to have a different vernacular name for kava.

The following chart (after Norton S.A. and Ruze, P.: "Kava dermopathy." *Journal of the American Academy of Dermatology*, 1994 July; 31, 1: 89-97) provides quite a comprehensive range of kava terminology from several of the dominant cultures:

English	Hawaiian	Tongan	Fijian
kava	'awa	kava	yaqona
kava bowl	kanoa	kumete	tanoa
kava cup	'apu 'awa	ipu kava	bilo
kava strainer	mau'u	tangai	ibo
chiefs	ali'i	hou'eiki	turaga
priest	kahuna	patele	-
server	kau'a	tou'a	tu yaqona
kava circle	-	'alofi	-
kava ceremony	hui'ava	'ilo kava	vakaturaga
dermopathy	mahuna	nafunafua	kani
intoxicated	'ona	kona	mateni
sacred (taboo)	kapu	tapu	tabu

In Hawaiian and some other languages, "kava" is not only a noun but also an adjective, meaning: "bitter," "sharp," "pungent," etc.

The most detailed account of the history of kava's nomenclature is provided by Vincent Lebot. The latest edition of *Kava: the Pacific Elixir* by Healing Arts Press (1997) is recommended for readers wishing to have further information on this topic.

Geography

To appreciate the geography of kava use it is desirable to have at hand a detailed map of the Pacific Ocean. The many small islands or island groups in which kava is grown and used are widely scattered throughout this enormous Ocean. A recent map is helpful, as the names of many islands have been changed in modern times, as have the names of countries in other parts of the world.

Oceania

The islands of the South Pacific may be conveniently grouped under the term *Oceania*. This covers a vast area, roughly bordered by New Guinea and Hawaii to the north and the eastern seaboard of Australia and New Zealand, to the south.

Further sub-divisions, going counterclockwise within Oceania, are: Micronesia, Melanesia and Polynesia. Just further to the northwest of Micronesia is Indonesia, which includes Bali, the stereotypical South Pacific community and prototype for the movie "South Pacific." However, the Balinese are quite unique in the region and seem to prefer fragrant incenses and tobaccos to kava. They are Hindu, while many of the other nations of this region are Buddhist.

Oceania, with its kava ceremonials, did not have the advanced religious practices developed in India or China. Indeed, people of Oceania were infamous for cannibalism, if that qualifies?

For convenience, refer to the accompanying cross-referenced lists, providing countries within regions and an alphabetical arrangement of countries, together with their respective region:

Region	Country
Micronesia	
	Ponape (Pohnpei)
	Kosrae (Kusaie)
Melanesia	
	Fiji
	Vanuatu (New Hebrides)
	New Guinea
	Solomon Islands
Polynesia	
	Hawaiian islands
	Marquesas Islands
	Society Islands (notably Tahiti)
	Samoa
	Tonga
	Wallis and Futuna
	Cook islands

Island		Region
Cook		Polynesia
Espiritu Santo	Vanuatu	Melanesia
Fiji		Micronesia
Hawaii		Polynesia
Kosrae (Kusaie)		Micronesia
Marquesas		Polynesia
New Guinea		Melanesia
Papua New Guinea		Melanesia

Pentecost	Vanuatu	Melanesia
Ponape (Pohnpei)		Micronesia
Samoa		Polynesia
Society		Polynesia
Solomon Islands		Melanesia
Tahiti	Society	Polynesia
Tanna	Vanuatu	Melanesia
Torres	Vanuatu	Melanesia
Vanuatu (New Hebrides)		
Melanesia		

Geographical Distribution of Kava Culture

Although kava is predominantly associated with Western Polynesia (Hawaii, Samoa, Tonga etc.) it is common to nearly all Pacific islands. The Maoris did take kava to New Zealand. Growing conditions were not right, however, so they made do with a close relative (Pipert excelsum), although it is not, apparently, suitable for a beverage. It has, however, been successfully integrated within their magico-religious rites. Easter Island, on the northern edge of New Zealand, was also too temperate for kava to flourish.

The largest land mass, Australia, was originally an exception to kava use throughout the Pacific. Quite recently, through inter-cultural exchanges with other indigenous people throughout Oceania, kava became known there as well. Numerous aboriginal tribes in Australia have had a serious addiction problem with certain Western products, much as the indigenous tribes of North America have had. This covers sniffing gasoline, as well as drinking alcohol, when available.

Unfortunately, rather than replacing other forms of substance abuse among Aboriginal cultures in Australia, kava was also abused. Aboriginal consumption of kava exceeded that of traditional users by fifty-fold!

Usage

Usage of kava has taken several forms over the centuries. Classically, it was taken in the form of a potent beverage, although the traditional preparation and nightly consumption have not found acceptance in the modern scheme of things, even in the South Seas. We will discuss these uses separately, as Traditional Preparation and Modern Preparation.

Traditional Preparation

The traditional, or Ancient, method has also come to be known as the "Tongan" method, although it seems to have been standard throughout the region before outside influences took over.

The Ancient Method involved using virgin girls or boys, who were in good health and had good teeth and masticatory ability. They were required to chew a wad of the fresh root until the fibers were thoroughly broken down. Although the enzymes are important to the process (rather as yeast is to the making of bread), it was considered ill-mannered to mix a large quantity of their saliva with the wad. Salivary enzymes assisted degradation to a fully intoxicating substance. The resultant liquid has been described as "a grayish-greenish-brown color."

The raw root possesses some potency, quite apart from having a very bitter taste, and the child would experience a numbing sensation and be unable to taste food, afterwards. This masticated mass, which may have tripled by weight, was then either placed on a banana leaf or spat directly into a kava bowl. Some ceremonial bowls would have been quite ornate, but for everyday use most people simply used half a coconut shell, which was, of course, in plentiful supply and recyclable.

Once three, or more, wads were ready, they would have been placed in the bowl and had water, or coconut milk, poured over them until it was judged that the desired strength had been reached. The pulp was then strained out through coconut palm fibers.

Most non-native people considered the Ancient Method pretty disgusting, and still do. Dutch explorers were the first Europeans to witness the ceremony, and a full one-hundred-fifty years later, Captain Cook and his crew left a number of records of their observations. Cook had this to say:

The manner of brewing, or preparing, the liquor is as simple as it is disgusting to a European and is thus: several people take of the root, or stem adjoining to the root and chew it into a kind of pulp, when they spit it out into a platter, or other vessel. ...When a sufficient quantity is done they mix with it a certain proportion of water and then strain the liquor through fibrous stuff and it is then fit for drinking which is always done immediately; it has a pepperish taste, rather flat and insipid and intoxicating." (1773)

Cook was the only member of his crew, as well as the first Westerner, adventurous enough to sample the brew, having witnessed how it was prepared!

Ceremonial

Traditionally, kava has been part of ceremonies for centuries, if not thousands of years. These events may be sub-divided into descending hierarchical order : on formal occasions; at regular meetings of VIP's; and at simpler gatherings of ordinary people—friends and families. Thus, three, in all.

In the first instance, the full, or "high kava" ceremony was used to greet Captain Cook, as well as Hilary Rodham Clinton more recently (1992). Guests are led to a platform; hosts are gathered around in a circle, sitting cross-legged. The ceremony begins with ritual chanting. Then a group of young men, dressed in ceremonial attire, bring in the bowl of kava and cups. From a kneeling posture, the host presents the first cup to the honored guest, who is instructed to drain it, without stopping. If this is duly accomplished everyone says *"a maca"* (pronounced "a matha"), declaring simply, "it is empty," and claps three times. The bearer returns to the bowl and serves the next most important person and so on.

The Queen of England and Hilary Clinton have been notable exceptions to this predominantly male activity. In some societies, kava drinking was restricted solely to royalty and priests. Gradually, while the social circle widened (After all, how could they restrict the use of something growing everywhere?), choice varieties of kava were still reserved for the high and mighty. Incidentally, a number of these nations have had notable Queens, as well as Kings, in their royal lineages, so it was not simply the fact that they were patriarchal societies that kept kava usage essentially limited to males.

Kava ceremonies today remain the most important cultural events for many of these nations, including Tonga and Fiji; just as they were at any time in the past. It may be said to form the quintessence of hospitality.

Kava is not just symbolized as a beverage. Cook received roots of kava from canoes sent out to greet his ship, taking the gift to be a sign of peace and friendship. When parties from within Oceania met one another, they would each give the other a gift of kava root. Kava root could seal a peace treaty. Indeed, on the island of Tanna within Vanuatu, a special type of kava is grown specifically for purposes of exchange. Nikava tapuga grows on the trunks of tree ferns, which seems to provide an especially attractive plant. When kava is used in a religious ceremony, it may not be drunk by those assembled. Instead, it is poured onto the ground.

In everyday life, kava gatherings are less formal and serve as social mixers, just like a "coffee club," or wine-tasting party. Most frequently, such gatherings are held at night and may continue until the next morning.

In Fiji, more extreme effects may be sought (often with malicious intent) so that kava is adulterated with another, more potent relative from the pepper family (Piper puberulum).

Modern Preparation

Today the fresh kava root is pounded, in a suitable container, into a fine powder. This may also have been the standard practice in Fiji at one time, where stones were used for pounding. Another early technique may have been scraping the root with the edge of a piece of coral, for example. Many of the islands of the South Pacific remain industrially quite primitive, so there is often a great deal of ingenuity present. The greatest source of machinery may well be the abandoned stock of the United States forces from the Second World War. This is not unlike the situation in the Eastern United States, where isolated, rural communities set up stills for moonshine distillation. The set-up may incorporate old automobile parts, like the radiator, for example. In Oceania, one popular pounding tool is the axle from a vehicle and the receptacle is likely to be a metal drum. Villages across the Pacific resound with this cacophony every evening ("tuki kava").

The ground powder is then placed in a fine-mesh bag (made from nylon stockings). Water is poured in a large bowl, and the bag is placed into the water and then worked with the fingers until the potency of the infusion achieves the desired color. The bag is thoroughly squeezed and set aside to be re-used later.

For a group of four or five people, a heaping one-quarter cup of powder and three pints of water is a good start for the first rendering. The same bag and powder can make at least another two or three bowls full. (Drinking as many as five and up to eight bowls would be a big night for a kava drinker. Even at the prices for the powder in the United States [$2 an ounce] this is an inexpensive treat.) Finally, hot water can be poured over the bag for a nightcap.

Singh has also recorded a third method which produces an especially potent brew. The process is similar to the regular infusion, using hot water, except that green stock is used. This variety might be used to put someone "under the table," rather like spiking the punch with vodka to get the party rolling.

Taste

Of course, different people have differing perceptions about any taste. To the South Sea Islanders, kava was certainly different tasting from water or coconut milk. A freshly dug root, without benefit of a thorough cleaning, would undoubtedly have an earthy-taste!

Emerson wrote that he enjoyed its "cooling, aromatic, numbing effect," finding relief from thirst while hiking through the woods (1903). This view is shared by a notable Polynesian physician practicing in New Zealand, Sir Peter Buck (Te Rangi Hiroa), who credits kava as being the "best drink for a tropical climate."

In the etymological section, we have noted how the word kava is, widely, synonymous with "sourness" and "bitterness." But, all of these considerations may be ignored by the typical Westerner who will consume kava in its encapsulated form, free of taste!

Chemistry

Kava may be classified as a psychoactive plant, in that it affects the central nervous system. Examples of such psychoactive plants cover a wide range from coffee—everyone's favorite morning breakfast drink to "jump start" the day—to others which are regarded in most Western countries, at least, as controlled substances or illegal street drugs, notably *cannabis* (marijuana).

With indigenous peoples, coca leaf is a stimulant, while the West is confronted by a much harsher and more intense derivative: cocaine. (At one time it was an ingredient in Coca Cola, which is where the name came from). Opium and heroin represent a similar continuum from the same Asiatic poppy.

Specifically, the action of kava (or how kava gets its kick) seems to be derived from kavalactones. These are contained within oil cells, which yield a greenish-yellow resin when released. The proportion of kavalactone concentrated in the roots can vary considerably, anywhere between three and twenty percent.

At first analysis there appeared to be at least nine compounds, known as kavalactones, kava pyrones, or kava alphapyrones. The three most important of these were thought to be:

kavain;
dihydrokavain (DHK); and
dihydromethysticin (DHM).

The major list today, which has now grown to fifteen, still includes three kavalactones, although the list membership has changed slightly. Vincent Lebot found that the first three (noted above) accounted for some seventy percent of the total:

1. Demetheoxyyangonin (DMY).
2. Dihydrokavain (DHK).
3. Yangoning (Y).
4. Kavain (K).
5. Dihydromethysticin (DHM).
6. Methysticin (M).

The anesthesia-like numbing effect seems to be associated with kavain. The kavalactones, generally, seem to have a distinct muscle-relaxing effect. They have a *direct* action on the muscles, rather than an indirect mechanism, via neurotransmitter signals, like other plant constituents. Kavalactones do not sedate the central nervous system, effectively blocking the neurotransmitter signals. Instead, muscles are relaxed, directly.

Method of Action

The kava drink is, variously: intoxicating, stimulating and psychoactive, providing a "natural high"; depending upon the strength and quantity consumed. Kava appears to have a mildly narcotic (i.e., sleep-inducing) action, which accounts for its current claim to fame in the West as "the calming herb." Although once frowned upon by missionaries, because of its associated intemperance, kava use now seems to be one reason why the stereotype, for people of the South Seas, is so relaxed and happy.

Rising doses of lactones depress the central nervous system at the level of the reticular formation of the brain stem and relax the skeletal muscles. Full consciousness is retained even after taking fatal doses. The drug is eliminated via the kidneys, but during its passage through the digestive system it produces numbing effects on all the membranes lining the stomach and bladder (just as it does in the mouth when chewing the raw root). Some European drugs capitalize upon this feature of kava kava to eliminate painful bladder syndromes. One such drug combines kava kava with pumpkin seeds and hops which have been traditionally employed, on their own, for prostate problems, for example.

In one study (by Garner and Klinger) the kava drink affected several parameters of vision. Specifically, it reduced near point of accommodation and convergence (explained below), also causing an increase in pupil diameter and a disturbance of the oculomotor balance. This is quite a concentrated amount of optical information for non-specialists, so we will elaborate on it for general readers.

Most middle-aged readers will wear glasses. They will have a comfortable point at which they can focus when reading a book. Without glasses, the main question will be whether their arms are long enough! This is because, as the eye's lens hardens with aging, it is less able to "accommodate," or focus upon, objects near at hand. Apparently kava is able to alter this, presumably through antioxidant action. Paradoxically, accommodation is usually accompanied by constriction of the pupil, although another feature identified for kava is increased pupil diameter. We have all tried to "squint" in order to aid accommodation to be able to read something that is not quite clear enough.

Convergence means that both eyes focus upon the same thing. Many people must turn their head to see something clearly, or sometimes close one eye, since one eye is usually dominant. (To determine which is the dominant eye, hold a thumb in line with a distant object, like a light switch. First use both eyes and then close each eye in turn. One eye, when used alone, will change the alignment of the thumb. The dominant eye will be the one that aligns the thumb in the same position as when both eyes are used.) It is noticeably difficult to align the thumb when using both eyes. In some people, it may be impossible to use both eyes together (strabismus) in which case a patch may be used to cover the dominant eye while working the "lazy" eye.

This cannot be successfully treated after early childhood. As the object being focused upon is closer, even the end of your nose, the eyes will eventually "cross." In some people this is a permanent condition which requires surgical correction.

Finally, if you are unaware of a link between vision and balance, close your eyes and then try to balance on one leg. Most people are very wobbly! It is interesting to conjecture that kava may have a role to play in ophthalmology, besides some rather bewildering visual changes (not unlike those affecting drivers under the influence of alcohol).

Effects

After early hesitancy, the reports from travelers and scientists on their experiences with kava have become quite abundant over the past half century, or so. They are also quite consistent, so just a few examples will suffice, further duplication being unnecessary.

Reports of kava's effects fall into several groups: the missionary describes kava as the brew of demon savages; even some natives are aware of some side effects; however most reports are highly favorable. We'll sample some views of each group:

The Puritanical outlook of the missionaries had no appreciation that kava was non-alcoholic but identified it with the heathen status and culture of Stone Age people. In order to save them for Christianity, they had to be rescued from such pursuits. William Ellis (c.1820) provided a typical description:

Under the unrestrained influence of their intoxicating draught, in their appearance and actions, they resembled demons more than human beings.

A native Hawaiian named Kaulilinoe, was quoted by Titcomb (1948):

There is no admiration for the body and face of a kava drinker whose eyes are sticky and whose skin cracks like...bark,...you will find your muscles and cords limp, the head feels weighted and the whole body too.

Ironically, in some societies the kava drinkers themselves wore the scaly skin, which often characterizes long-term use, as a badge of honor. Once again, this is much like the different cultural perspectives that exist regarding tattoos, which were also common in the South Seas. Traditional methods were exceedingly painful, and tattooing often covered the whole body. Both the pain and the extent of coverage would have been too much for most non-native people to bear. However, within the South Seas it was a tradition. (Just a few years ago no one could have predicted the resurgence of interest in tattooing, even piercing, in modern Western societies. Perhaps there is some primal need that many of us can no longer relate to?)

Lemert succinctly summarized the dominant effects of kava (1967): The head is affected pleasantly; you feel friendly; kava quiets the mind.

Addiction to Kava?

Overall, there seems to be general agreement on the following points:

- A few cupfuls of kava may provide a "high," or state of euphoria of short duration, accompanied by tranquillity and friendliness.
- Unlike alcohol, there is no hangover and the mind remains clear. A typical serving size for kava is around five ounces (or 150 mls), so even three cups would still be under the traditional pint of English beer. A perfectly reasonable serving, even if it were as alcoholic as beer!
- Like alcohol, it is soporific, although it causes calmness and relaxation, with enhanced mental activity and promotes a deep, dreamless sleep.

This outline paints a far better picture for kava's effects than the scenes of contemporary violence perpetrated by the "lager louts" who follow British soccer teams; or the broken families abandoned by gin-drinking mothers in London (earning for gin the name "Mother's Ruin" in Cockney slang). While some experts seem to suggest that the French habit of drinking wine with dinner is probably beneficial to health, there can be "too much of any good thing"—each major city in the U.S. has a "Skid Row" littered with the helpless bodies of "winos." Examples of alcohol abuse abound throughout the world.

Abuse is partly a matter of the dosage and the other part, of course, is the person who takes the dose. In the Western world it currently seems unlikely that the introduction of kava will create a "Skid Row" festooned with kava abusers. Indeed, most people will consume kava as a capsule, or standardized tincture. It is, as such, a health supplement, devoid of any social gatherings or connotations—however beneficial they may be. Many of those people will be industrious, seeking some relaxation and a good night's sleep. Compared with alcohol and prescription drugs, kava is almost devoid of serious problems.

In Australia, however, the situation is entirely different. Kava drinking was imported to Aboriginal communities to replace other forms of substance abuse. The consumers, however, were already "lost souls," in many respects. Consequently, the pattern became for them to consume up to fifty-times the amount habitually consumed by kava drinkers in traditional societies. (It takes some effort to consume a gallon of anything!) There are fears that kava drinking will be yet another health and social problem for these communities.

These abusers are after oblivion, not improved health. They would not readily switch from the kava drink to a capsule, if it were to be offered to them. Kava, in terms of an herbal supplement for indicated health conditions, is an entirely different matter from kava in the traditional form of a beverage; or the consumption of kava within an at-risk community, like that of the Aborigines.

A major distinction between alcohol and kava, repeated time and time again in the literature, is the fact that kava drinkers awaken alert and refreshed; which is in marked contrast to the "hangover" of an alcoholic.

A common sense approach, like that applied with many different beverages, should prevail with regard to kava. For example, it is quite common to purchase apple juice, even for babies. However, fermented apple juice, or cider, can be quite potent and does wreak havoc with the central nervous system when taken in excess over a long period of time. The distinction is quite simple. It is a non-issue, when shopping at the market, which product to purchase and what is a reasonable amount for even a baby to drink.

Another factor, inhibiting the expansion of kava drinking and abuse in Western countries is that the concentrate from which the beverage can be made retails at around $90 an ounce and must be shipped from either Vanuatu, or Hawaii. Appropriate usage of kava is discussed further in the following sections which deal with kava for specific health conditions (see Chapters 4, 5, 6 and 7).

In summary, Lebot has reminded us that in spite of its associations, kava is, in fact: "non-fermented, non-alcoholic, non-opioid (and) non-hallucinogenic..."

The Scientific Evidence So Far

The reported effects of kava inspired chemical investigations that have occupied scientists for almost one-hundred-fifty years! The first step is always to isolate the biologically active compounds and then to synthesize them, allowing the product to be manufactured consistently, just like aspirin, for a specific effect. Yangonin, for example, although isolated in 1874 was not synthesized until 1960.

Chemical Composition

The first scientific investigations, on record, of the chemical composition of kava, were done by Gobley (1860) and Cuzent (1861), at almost the same time, and isolated the same substance. This crystalline substance was named variously: *kavahine*, *kavakin* and *kavatin*, and has now become firmly established as *methysticin*. Kava pills and other products, including an oleoresin, an alcohol extract and a syrup were sold by German herbal stores around that time.

The next kavalactone was isolated in 1874 by Nolting and Koop, but it was named by Lewin a few years later (1886): *yangonin*. Dihydromethysticin (DHM) followed from the work of Winzheimer (1908).

Between 1914 and 1933 Borsche undertook an intense study of kava, publishing fourteen papers, essentially adding two additional kavalactones—*kawain* and *dihydrokawain* (DHK)—to the three that already existed.

While some alkaloid content was suspected, it was too unstable before 1979 when R. M. Smith isolated *pipermethysticine*. While present in small amounts in stems and roots, it is a major constituent of the kava leaves.

As more advanced equipment became available (moving from spectrophotometry to chromatography and gas liquid chromatography [GLC]), the accuracy of previous analysis was improved. By 1973 Shulgin was able to rank the proportion of the major components in kava:

Major: dihydrokawain, kawain and methysticin.
Minor: dehydromethysticin, dihydromethysticin, desmethoxyyangonin, yangoning and flavakawin-A.
Trace: flavakawin-B, methoxynoryangoning and methoxyyangonin.

Duve (1984), using GLC, established assays to evaluate the effectiveness of various extraction procedures as well as evaluate the stability of the constituents during storage as powder.

Duffield (1989) discovered previously unknown trace elements, using methane chemical ionization gas chromatography/mass spectroscopy.

Thus, the chemical analysis is available and it remains for pharmacologists to match the particular kavalactone, or kavalactones, with the appropriate illness for an effective remedy.

Pharmacology

Historical Perspectives
Early pharmacological evaluation of kava pyrones is now considered to be only of historical interest because of the low level of sophistication involved in such procedures. Only limited amounts of major compounds were available for Lewin, for example.

By 1924, Schubel concluded that kava resin: had a weak sleep-inducing action, paralyzed sensory nerves, and could first stimulate and then paralyze smooth muscles. Schubel confirmed that kava extract had an increased potency when activated by human saliva. Presumably, the saliva was able to reduce the starch component (43%) thereby concentrating the proportion of kavalactones.

Schubel worked with isolated kavalactones (methysticin and yangonin) but could not reproduce the activity of the whole. In 1933, Borsche also conceded that none of the isolated kavalactones available to them (methysticin, dihydromethysticin, yangonin, kawain and dihydrokawain) could achieve the effects reputed for the crude preparation.

However, later researchers were able to reproduce well-known effects, like sleep, with DHK (dihydrokawain).

Just after the Second World War, Meyer initiated the modern era of kava research at Freiburg University in the beautiful Black Forest region of southern Germany. He found that kavalactones produced the following effects: analgesic, anticonvulsant, muscle relaxant and sedative. Meyer demonstrated that kavalactones produced muscular relaxation in all laboratory animals. The South Sea islanders hadn't been imagining these things for thousands of years after all!

Hansel and Beiersdorff (1959 in Germany) successfully used both DHK and DHM to induce sleep in mice and rats when administering the extracts as an emulsion via stomach tube.

Given the earlier concentration on water-soluble pyrones, Buckley and his colleagues investigated the water-soluble fractions obtained from kava by steam distillation (1967). Two distillates were relatively free of pyrones but exhibited similar effects, albeit at higher doses. Muscular relaxation occurred, as well as anti-serotonin activity.

Contemporary Issues
Even though willow bark (aspirin) was used for thousands of years before its chemical pathways were

unraveled, the scientific method generally requires that at least some effort be made to isolate the precise mechanism which defeats the disease process. Allopathic medicine just doesn't like to admit it doesn't have all the answers!

Finding and producing a "magic bullet" can prove to be two ends of the same stick, or involve entirely separate entities. A natural product, like kava, can be studied to identify traditional uses. It can then be analyzed to see if there is a compound that is consistent with contemporary chemistry and pharmacology. Sometimes there will be a match. The pharmacologists may have found what they were looking for! More likely, the chemistry will take some time to catch-up with the "folk uses." In the meantime, some scientists will advocate the herb at face value because it does have unique substances, although the pathway hasn't been identified; while others will seek to suppress its use until these pathways have been elucidated fully. The clinical trials may take a totally different direction from traditional uses, possibly restricted by the known metabolic pathways.

Matters become more complicated if the preparation (in our case kava) does not achieve the full effect that is desired, by itself. Indeed, as in the Traditional Chinese system of herbal medicine, more and more products are combining kavalactones with other herbs, for a synergistic effect, beyond anything achievable with either herb, individually (as the dictum goes: "The whole exceeds the sum of the individual parts"). The combination of kava and valerian for insomnia is a notable example. Another is the use of kava with St. John's Wort for mental well being. In these cases, an established remedy is given an additional boost (potentiated) by the use of kava or an isolated kavalactone. This may be likened to a "shotgun" approach.

Similarly, many naturopathic practitioners are suspicious of isolated products, preferring the natural synergy of the whole (as in [w]holism). Murray for example, a well-known naturopath and author, has commented that: "The whole complex of kavalactones, together with other compounds found in kava, produce greater pharmacological activity."

Klohs during the mid-1950s could not obtain the same results from any of the crystalline compounds that he could from the ground root, or crude extract of kava. He postulated a synergetic action from their combination.

Cynically, viewing the pharmaceutical industry from a naturopathic perspective, the whole plant cannot be patented. Also, the herbal product may be used without a prescription. Therefore, the financial investment is restricted, as there is no likelihood of a high return. Nonetheless, if the herb (kava) effects a cure and enough people know about it, the whole medical-industrial complex (allopathic physicians, pharmaceutical manufacturers, pharmacies and hospitals) is bypassed! If the market for a pharmaceutical is lost, the financial losses can be colossal, affecting the security of the entire parent company. In the case of kava, its role, with or without St. John's Wort, seems likely to conflict with Prozac.

Certainly, pharmacologists have not been active as long as chemists yet their results so far seem to largely corroborate traditional observations.

Duffield and Jamieson, in New South Wales (Australia), have more recently (1990) indicated that while kava may provide the same benefit as a prescription sedative, like Valium, it achieves this effect via a different pathway. Whereas Valium (one of the world's most frequently prescribed drugs, together with fellow benzodiazepines, e.g. Halcion) is taken up by particular receptors in the brain (known as GABA [gamma-aminobutyric acid] receptors) which promote sedation, kavalactones do not bind in the same way.

Jussogie observed that effects of kavapyrones were due to an increase in the number of binding sites, rather than to a change in affinity. When kavapyrones were included together with pentobarbital they produced a more than additive, i.e., a synergetic effect. They seem to target the limbic system, which is known as the seat of the emotions.

Kava drinkers have traditionally been friendly and peaceful, unlike the aggressiveness of many beer drinkers. However, the animal models studied for kava's effects do not have sophisticated enough brains to identify the precise mechanisms involved. Gleitz found a fast and specific inhibition of sodium channels in the rat brain by kavain. It may affect the master mechanism of the brain, within the limbic system, thereby modifying the receptor domain itself, rather than simply the binding-site.

Traditionally, kava drinkers have been distinguished by their hearing acuity during sleep, and every effort was made to maintain silence around them. Some visual enhancement has also been reported (Garner and Klinger). Therefore, several major areas and functions of the brain and spinal cord seem to be involved, far beyond a few receptor sites. Kava, therefore, does not merely change the channel on your TV set, so-to-speak, it provides a big screen with stereo, plus digital pictures and sound!

Similarly, accepting that kava provided pain relief, researchers looked at the typical opioid receptors. (Even athletes obtain pain relief via this mechanism, via their beta-endorphins, which makes human beings so vulnerable to opiates. The receptors are already in place!) Leaving morphine behind, studies looked at other pain models, for which aspirin and nonsteroidal anti-inflammatory drugs (like Advil, or Motrin, i.e., ibuprofen) have proven to be ineffective. Kava worked, therefore, differently from accepted varieties of pain relievers, and without any of their side-effects (addiction, gastrointestinal disturbances, internal bleeding, etc.).

Another interesting finding (Kinzler and Lehman), this time with respect to anxiety, was that when compared to standard, prescription anxiolytic drugs, kava did not exhibit any loss of effectiveness over time. Patients did not build up resistance, or tolerance, towards it.

Finally, kava also proved to be effective in cases of stroke, limiting the infarct area in models of focal cerebral ischemia (a loss of blood supply to a specific region of the brain). Animals receiving kava did not sustain such large losses of brain cells as control animals. Hence kava is being combined with Ginkgo Biloba by some manufacturers to potentiate their effect on the blood circulation within the brain.

All in all, kavalactones have not only proven their efficacy, they have done so in superior fashion. They have not only been proven to work effectively, they work in different ways to provide greater benefits with fewer side effects over a longer period of time.

The Politics and Economics of Kava

Several plants, some with therapeutic benefits, exist in a nebulous state of legitimacy, and still provide a large cash income. Tobacco is basically legal, and even marijuana has been legalized (in California for example) so far as terminally ill patients are concerned. Tobacco is sold quite inexpensively on the ordinary market, although this may increase with the compensatory fines or tax burdens in some countries. Marijuana, like cocaine and opium, commands high prices on the "Black Market."

So, where does kava fit in? Do we have the studies to legitimize medical use? Should it be a drug only available on prescription? How likely is it to be abused? What economic interests will seek to establish themselves, politically?

Sponsoring Studies

Due to the fact that there is no patent process available for natural plant products, potential revenues from such products are reduced. Patented medicines can be sold at much higher cost than non-patented medicine. Consequently, while funds are available for the type of studies required for approval of a synthetic drug (at least by the FDA in the United States), limited financial resources are available for natural product studies. Hence, natural products are usually criticized for this "oversight."

Although kava already has a significant amount of literature, clinical studies are difficult to undertake and often depend upon the availability of funding from some vested interest. We can recognize such factors at work with studies undertaken on tobacco and nicotine, sponsored by tobacco companies; as well as studies on sweeteners sponsored by manufacturers of aspartame products. (It is now becoming evident that the powerful tobacco lobbies were able to suppress evidence, on the one hand, and even develop special varieties of tobacco, on the other, to elevate the nicotine content of their cigarettes, rendering them even more addictive, thereby maintaining sales in a shrinking market. Veteran smokers would have a more difficult time giving up the habit, while any new converts would be addicted more quickly, with a greater likelihood of a high consumption rate over a long period of time.)

In Australia, one study, sponsored by the alcohol industry, looked for negative associations for kava drinkers within the Aboriginal communities. Of course, such associations were not difficult to find. Kava drinkers showed a number of physical ill-effects, including: dermopathy, underweight, low blood values and generally poor health status, including lung function.

The Australian Issue

The Australian situation is quite unique and merits a thorough review. As noted earlier, kava drinking was imported to Aboriginal communities to replace other forms of substance abuse, but soon became a problem in its own right. Kava drinkers here consumed up to fifty times the amount habitually used in traditional societies.

Following the study sponsored by the alcohol industry (mentioned above), removing kava from the scene was recommended as a way to improve the health status of Aboriginal communities. Of course, the unstated goal was to secure the market for the alcohol industry. This eventually came out and discredited the report.

When missionaries had previously removed kava from the scene, or driven it underground, some Cook islanders learned to brew their own alcohol from fermented orange juice, which they substituted for kava. Ceremonial use of this beverage was given the same name, *tumu nu*, as had been used for the former kava ceremony.

The state of devastation in Aboriginal communities is very similar to that within the United States on Native American reservations. Both groups of indigenous people also show a remarkable affinity for substance abuse while exhibiting a low tolerance to it. Hence, if there is any likelihood of an attendant side effect, or negative consequence for their action, they will more than likely suffer from it at rates well beyond those in the non-native community, especially. Such morbid consequences range from being drunk on a small quantity of alcohol, to amputation associated with diabetes, and on to high mortality rates from traumatic events, including drunk driving.

Under such dire circumstances, the actual substance of abuse has little relevance. It is difficult to deny access to every product which can be abused, or to protect people from themselves, since this is "self-abuse." Desperate people will switch from alcohol, to gasoline, to paint, to glue, to hair spray and so on. If they can't find it at the store they may find it on the prairie, like peyote or certain mushrooms.

Kava *can* be abused and can induce negative health consequences. However, the level of consumption required is colossal. It requires a nightly excess over many months, if not years, to develop the dermopathy. The hopeless social context seen among the Australian Aborigines has never occurred in the South Pacific.

Approval Process

Most of the research on kava has arrived by way of Europe, where kava has received formal approval. The approval process in Europe has been far less arduous than in the United States.

Plants with traditional uses do not require approval to the same extent as a new synthetic drug product, which can take several years and tens of millions of dollars. The backlash from this is that the allopathic community will look down upon a product which does not have the standard reports from double-blind, randomized, controlled trials accompanying it. They overlook the fact that the majority of the pharmaceutical products at their disposal fall short of this standard, also.

A plant product may be imported and sold, but it won't be protected by patent and cannot command the same price level as typical pharmaceutical products. This means a lower potential return on investment, which reduces that investment. The first thing to go will be the patient trial. Indeed, the product is not likely to be prescribed very much in allopathic practice.

Conflict of Interest

As the example of Australia revealed, without government funding for an independent laboratory, the negative study on kava in Aboriginal communities was funded by alcohol interests with an ulterior motive—i.e., to suppress potential competition—

rather than by the kava importers themselves, who would have had a direct financial interest. Any "scientific" studies in the West, following standard pharmaceutical protocols, are likely to be few and far between. The significance of this depends upon one's point of view.

On one hand, no kava product would have an official seal of approval and be suitable for prescription by allopathic physicians. On the other hand, official approval would place it beyond the reach of naturopathic physicians or the traditional over-the-counter sales of herbal products directly to natural health consumers.

Quite recently (and throughout the past few decades following the U.S. Surgeon General's warning on cigarette packages) we have been able to observe (often first hand via live television coverage of U.S. Congressional hearings) how a rich and powerful lobby like that of the tobacco industry, will suppress negative studies and promote positive studies with "pseudo science." The tobacco industry has gone so far as to publicly deny, under oath, any association between nicotine and addiction, or (until recently) acknowledge a relationship between smoking and illness. This "ice castle" is now melting around them, however, and U.S. tobacco product manufacturers are paying billions of dollars of compensation.

Along similar lines, is the face-off between aspartame, a highly lucrative synthetic sweetener, and stevia, an herbal alternative. Most people still won't have heard of stevia, and those who have would have been unable to obtain it for several years because powerful interests were able to have its importation banned.

Like the tobacco companies, the aspartame producer suppressed negative studies and promoted their own pseudo-research, which claimed not to have found any negative associations for consumers of their product. On the other hand, the U.S. FDA received, and continues to receive, more complaints about aspartame than for any other product. Who are we to believe?

Kava Cultivation

The recent upsurge of interest from Europe and the U.S. has boosted kava cultivation throughout the South Pacific: Fiji, Hawaii, New Guinea, Samoa and Tahiti, among others. In fact the principal country, so far as kava is concerned, is Vanuatu (specifically its major island, Espiritu Santo), although its name may not be widely recognized. Like many countries which have gained independence from their colonial masters, it used to be the New Hebrides.

In Vanuatu, kava is the third-ranking crop export, behind coconut (termed *copra*) and cocoa. In Fiji, kava is second only to sugarcane. However, domestic users still account for the majority of crops in each country. Vanuatu cultivates the greatest amount of kava, and its product has the reputation for the highest potency.

Today, there are kava bars on some islands, rather like the public houses of England, except that they are more like a beach hut than a distinctive landmark.

Scores of these bars, Nakamals, exist in Vanuata, for example. The primary use of kava by the locals is a social drink, each evening. That kava has survived the ravages of colonialism and withstood the onslaught of international brewery companies, says something for its merits.

Export Markets

Kava was never used everywhere throughout the region of Oceania, and missionaries further limited the extent of kava's domain. However, the void was usually filled by alcohol, most of which was imported. Today, many newly independent governments are looking at ways to improve their situation. Kava represents a possible cash crop, as well as a means of replacing alcohol imports and stemming alcohol abuse.

Farther afield, but still along the Pacific rim (or "Ring of Fire"), where kava will not grow, expatriates create a ready market. By 1990, Australia, New Zealand and the United States accounted for an estimated ten tons per annum.

The U.S. herbal market has been flourishing since then, and kava products seem likely to gain a substantial segment of the market for substances to relieve stress and promote calmness and tranquillity.

Pharmaceutical markets for kava have become firmly established in France and Germany, although they have different requirements. The French import thirty tons of dried kava rootstock and process it into an alcohol extract. Early methods of extraction yielded as little as four grams from one kilo (about 1.5 gms per pound) of rootstock. As we have already noted, Germany takes fifty tons annually, largely to become standardized herbal extract. The sales of this extract amount to eight million dollars yearly.

Income

It is also important to consider the "micro-economics," how much income the individual farmer can expect from raising kava. Lebot has provided quite an extensive analysis from several viewpoints based upon figures reported by the Fijian Department of Agriculture and Ministry of Primary Industries (1984). At the time of that report, kava commanded the highest price per kilogram of any cash crop, up to $4.50, while sugar, cassava, and rice fetched less than a quarter of that price. However, the area planted and the yield still placed sugar at the top by a factor of four in comparison with kava: $75 and $18 million, respectively.

The individual farmer received approximately $25 per working day for his efforts, most of which occurred in the first year of the four year cycle, in clearing and preparing the land. Indeed the first year may require 176 days of work, whereas the harvesting, in the fourth year, may only need 28 days.

Since value is added at each stage, it is likely that the islands will undertake more sophisticated processing as time goes on and revenues increase. Most promising is an instant, ready-to-use powder, which would make a kava beverage as accessible as tea or coffee, anywhere in the world. In particular, qualitatively, certain varieties and parts will be selected for the different markets: beverage, pharmaceutical etc., so that purchasers will be assured of a consistent product. The pharmaceutical companies are interested in the kavalactone content, regardless of the palatability. Consumers of the traditional beverage, on the other hand, seek subtle flavors and physiological effects.

Herbs and the Nervous System

Researcher Titcomb provided an erudite summary for this chapter (1948) when he wrote how Hawaiians found that kava was essential to good health. They used it to soothe the nerves, induce relaxation, for sleep and to counteract fatigue. In so doing, he marked out the antithesis of our modern lifestyle! We are "on edge," we are stressed, we're hyperactive, we're insomniacs and totally devoid of energy. We can almost write our own prescription for kava, if the Hawaiians were right!

Herbs, like Kava, are indeed useful for stress and other anxiety-related disorders (hence the group designation as: anxiolytics). To that end, it is important to arrive at a precise understanding of the nature of stress and nervous disorders. First of all, although these conditions are presented individually, it does not mean that they are necessarily distinct from one another. Indeed, many occur together and even change, back and forth. Details of a number of relevant anxiety and stress disorders are provided in the latter part of this chapter to help the reader identify where they might fit in. But first we need to look at the working of the central nervous system.

Understanding the Central Nervous System

Conventional biochemistry has provided in-depth (but by no means complete) information on the workings of the central nervous system. We have identified neurotransmitters and their receptor sites, and can now exploit these by powerful drugs that follow the same pathways. In so doing, these drugs can increase the availability of a certain substance. On the other hand, by occupying a receptor site with a pseudo-substance, thereby effectively blocking them to a certain chemical, these drugs can cause a reduction of the level of a particular substance in the body.

Examples of such drug categories include: monoamine oxidase inhibitors (MAO's) and selective serotonin reuptake inhibitors (SSRI's) such as fluoxetine hydrochloride (Prozac). MAO's are usually the second-choice to tricyclic antidepressants because of a preponderance of side effects. Tricyclic drugs (like Amitryptiline) have been compared to the herb St. John's Wort in a number of trials.

Still, the success rate for dealing with depression by using drugs is often low, while the probability of side effects is quite high. For example, St. John's Wort, in preliminary findings, is promising (like many other herbal treatments) to be just the opposite: exhibiting a high success rate with a low incidence of side effects.

It may be too easy to assign herbs like kava and St. John's Wort to the same pathways as prescription drugs in order to satisfy certain factions. Certainly, even if the pathway is basically the same, the advantages and disadvantages are clearly different. Phytopharmaceuticals do not, simply, take over from existing pharmaceuticals. A paradigm shift must take place, so that the patient's needs are viewed differently and the selection of herbal treatments is undertaken from a whole new perspective.

The Nervous System from the Holistic Perspective

The holistic view has always been somewhat different from the allopathic view. Just as the patient is the focus, rather than the disease, this view appreciates that the mind (or central nervous system) does not operate in isolation from the body. Mainstream medicine is only now appreciating this fact, as Mind-Body Medicine, or with the poly-syllabic title of "psycho-neuro-immunology." The key feature in herbal treatment, one of the primary approaches within the holistic perspective, is balance, just like in Traditional Chinese Medicine, in which a balance of the two essential life-energies—the Yin and Yang—is sought.

With respect to the nervous system, the autonomic nervous system is sub-divided (for the convenience of a physiological understanding) into functional categories: sympathetic and para-sympathetic.

The Sympathetic Nervous System

The sympathetic nervous system exerts control over our functional abilities, including our reaction to stress (the instinctual "fight or flight" mechanism). It has a very close link to areas of the endocrine system (e.g., the adrenal-pituitary axis), which serves to further exemplify the futility of trying to separate these two systems in clinical practice. Blood supply, glucose levels and heart rate are regarded as being under sympathetic control. It is said that people experienced in meditation are able to deliberately alter these functions.

Parasympathetic Nervous System

The parasympathetic nervous system basically has the opposite action of the sympathetic nervous system. It primes our body for growth and regeneration. It is more subtle and operates mostly at night, during rest and recovery. If the sympathetic system becomes too powerful, heart disorders and diabetes often develop. If the parasympathetic system dominates, the person will be cold and lethargic.

Nervine Herbs

As we have seen, the nervous system can be overactive or underactive and there are herbal remedies to treat accordingly. Herbs which effect the "nervous system" are generally called "nervines." Specific herbs will act in a particular way, much like their pharmaceutical counterparts: restorative, antidepressant, etc. Nervine Relaxants calm the system; Nervine Stimulants stimulate it; Nervine Restoratives, or Tonics, tone the nervous system, keeping it in good working order.

Nervine Relaxants

The Nervine Relaxants are the closest natural alternative to tranquilizers. Care should be taken, however, not to go overboard, into a state of over-sedation.

In addition to Kava, there are other nervines like Chamomile, Hops, Lavender, Passion Flower and Valerian which act on the nervous system to calm and relax. Some of these herbs act on more than one part of the body to promote relaxation. As we all know from a long hot bath, a relaxed body encourages a relaxed mind. Kava has a dual action, working both on the nervous system and the muscle tissue as does Valerian.

Experts believe that the effects of kava are due to kava alphapyrones, which confer calmness and relaxation with enhanced mental activity without any of the side-effects of drugs or alcohol. The full chemical pathway for most of these herbs remains to be discovered. Some interact with the monoamine oxidase (MAO) system to prolong the action of certain neurotransmitters.

Nervine Stimulants

Stimulant herbs promote sympathetic functions. Cayenne, for example, is a nervine stimulant.

Nervine Restoratives

Nervous restoratives are medicines which tend to restore fine balance in autonomic function, either stimulating or restorative. One beauty of herbs is that they tend to provide whichever action the body requires (the term "Adaptogen" was developed specifically for ginseng for this very reason). They restore the normal balance, whether "up" or "down," or sympathetic or parasympathetic, respectively. Some herbs are renowned as "nutritives" for their ability to rebuild nerve tissue.

Anxiety and Related Disorders

Anxiety

Anxiety is a state of uneasiness, characterized by worry, apprehension or fear. It begins as a normal reaction to a threat against emotional or physical well being. Anxiety is usually accompanied by physical sensations. It becomes problematic when it persists, or is not readily attributable to a known cause, and interferes with normal daily functioning.

Anxiety attacks may provoke any of the following symptoms:

- Breathlessness
- Choking sensation
- Dizziness
- Fainting
- Hyperventilation

- Intense feeling of apprehension or fear
- Pupils widely dilated
- Racing or pounding chest
- Spasms of the stomach
- Tremors

Clinical trials in Germany used D, L-kavain, a purified kavalactone, at a dose of 44 milligrams daily. Scholing conducted a formal trial of eight-four patients who displayed symptoms of anxiety. Kavain improved a number of measurable factors, including: memory, reaction time and vigilance.

Lindenberg, directly compared kava with the pharmaceutical, oxazepam (a member of the more familiar group of Benzodiazepines) which is still available in the U.S. under the brand name: "Serax". The kavain group scored just as well as the oxazepam group but was free from the known complications of this family of drugs, including addiction and side effects, such as: dizziness, drowsiness and even hepatitis!

Psychological Disorders

Kinzler undertook a study with patients suffering from anxiety syndrome (1991). The Hamilton Anxiety Scale provided the standard. After completion of the month-long study, the kava extract group (100 mg t.i.d.) had a reduction in their anxiety, feelings of nervousness and physical manifestations (including: chest pains, dizziness, gastric irritation, heart palpitations and headache). The group was free of side effects and the degree of change reached statistical significance (it was totally objective and not subjective or the result of chance).

Lehman (1996) has published the most recent report on the subject of nervous disorders (specifically: states of anxiety, tension and excitedness). Patients received 100 mg of 70% standardized kava extract three times daily, over one month. He concluded that this kava protocol was clinically effective in reducing these states. In marked contrast to most pharmaceutical studies, no side effects were noted during this study.

This looks very positive, just as the Hawaiians had discovered, empirically, thousands of years ago. "But what if..." the kava puts you into a dream-like state throughout the day? Certainly, some authorities have warned against prescribing kava for patients who are already suffering from depression. It may deepen it for them. However, for those who are highly-stressed and may end up with a nervous breakdown, or become clinically depressed, kava seems to provide just the right amount of stimulation and mood enhancement.

Two studies, by Herberg and Munte, addressed these problems. To test whether kava would be associated with depressed mental function and/or impaired driving skills, they recorded event-related potentials with an EEG (electro-encephalograph) for a recognition memory test, consisting of words presented visually. The subjects taking kava showed a slightly increased word recognition rate and recorded a larger difference on the EEG tracings. Recommended levels of kava did not promote sedation but did stimulate mental acuity.

When Van Vleet worked with pigeons (1938) he discovered that kava extract had an enhanced effect when it was given as an emulsion (lecithin and water). More recent work has confirmed lecithin's importance in brain function, via some of its phospholipids, notably phosphatidylserine (PS) and phosphatidyl- choline (PC). This would lead someone to the conclu- sion that taking a blend of kava and lecithin, would constitute a "smart nutrient"! Expect to see just such a product by the next time you go to your local health food store!

Overall, then, there is ample scientific support for the popular tradition of kava as the "calming herb" of the South Pacific.

Stress

More and more Westerners are confronted by anxiety, burnout, depression and fatigue, which seem to be the price we pay for our complex, highly-stressed lifestyles. We all experience stress to a greater or lesser degree. A certain amount of stress is actually good for us. It is normal and even stimulating. However, an excessive amount can be harmful; more so when stress accumulates to a point where it starts to take over our lives.

There are all sorts of reasons why people suffer from stress. A change in a person's environment can cause it; it can be related to work, bereavement, or one's lifestyle; it can be brought on by something as simple as standing in a slow-moving line, or sitting in a traffic jam. Stress may be caused by worry: about business, or unpaid bills, or even having a disagreement with your significant other, or next door neighbor.

Mental stress affects the way our bodies function, but physical sources of stress must also be mentioned, which further compound the problem. Poor ventilation, smoking, uncomfortably high or low room temperatures, atmospheric pollution, the effects of electromagnetic waves from domestic, factory and office equipment (e.g., VDT's, microwave ovens, overhead power cables), chemical food additives and poor nutrition all take their toll on the modern person's ability to cope with their environment.

To the body, the cause of stress is unimportant—its reactive, or coping mechanisms, or what the experts call a "fight or flight response," are the same. The body prepares itself for the expected danger and increases its production of chemicals called stress hormones. This may result in rapid breathing, a heightening of all the senses, tensing of muscles and a rush of adrenaline.

Contrary to what we may think, stress is not a twentieth-century invention. It has been with us since the dawn of time. Imagine a Stone-Age man venturing out of his cave in his daily search for food. He is feeling calm, enjoying the moment. As he breathes in the cool air, a sense of well being envelops him. He pauses for a minute and takes in the scenery around him, totally relaxed. Suddenly, his serenity is smashed by a crashing noise in the forest. He shifts dramatically from a state of relaxation to one of tension, his heart pounding and muscles taut. As the rustling in the woods comes closer, his mouth becomes dry and a cold shiver goes down his spine. He looks around, picks up a sharp piece of rock, ready for the enemy. His mind instinctively considers the options: must he fight or can he flee?

Now the enemy comes into full view. It is a mountain lion which quickly disappears into the undergrowth upon sensing the presence of the caveman. As for the latter, his breathing eases and he returns to the relative safety of his cave. There are no clocks or deadlines providing his stress, only survival. Does he have fuel for the fire? Water to drink? Food to eat? Skins for warmth? A mate? He has survived this round. Perhaps he needs to dig a trap for the lion, or hunt it down, so that it won't surprise him again.

Compare that scenario to the twentieth century man who is easing his way into morning traffic on the freeway. Did he remember to fuel up? Is it time for his oil change? Is he going to spill his coffee? Will someone allow him on? Is traffic running smoothly? Will he be late? Did he remember everything in his briefcase? As he sits in the barely-moving traffic, he feels his anxiety build: he's worried about being late, which will upset lunch and his afternoon schedule and he's still preoccupied with yesterday's deal that still hadn't closed. He'll have to miss his workout again. (Oh well, that's a good excuse. He doesn't enjoy it anyway.)

He finally arrives at the office twenty minutes late, to find that his boss has left a threatening memo on his desk. His anxiety becomes palpable, as his heart pounds and muscles become taut. His mouth becomes dry, his head throbs and a cold shiver runs down his spine. He looks around, sights a golf club and resists the impulse to smash something with it. Instead he slams his office door, thumps his fist down hard on his desk, hurting himself in the process and, in pain and resignation, reaches into his desk drawer for a few aspirin...better, make it three: "It's going to be one of those days," he sighs to himself. The concrete jungle isn't far removed from the first scenario, after all, is it?

Emotional trauma is the most common source of stress and the well-known Holmes-Rahe stress-factor rating scale lists bereavement, divorce, relationship problems and financial difficulties as familiar examples. Even our kids are stressed, with school, homework, grades, over-loaded schedules, and little time to just "hang-out." Nowadays, instead of fleeing, or fighting, we tend to "stew" in our own chemical soup, which is why we suffer so much more than our ancestors. Once they had reached safety, or won the battle, the stress was over. They could go to sleep and wake up refreshed the next day. (Doesn't this sound exactly like a description of the traditional kava drinkers!)

Short term stress will not usually cause any long term problems. However, repetitive stress will gradually weaken the immune system and deplete the body of essential nutrients. Even trivial everyday problems will suddenly become unmanageable and grow out of all proportion. The person may feel tense, moody and hyperactive just sitting and watching a TV show. Over the long term, the damage is potentially serious. High blood pressure, high blood cholesterol levels and heart disease are all stress-related diseases.

Whether it is caused by physical or emotional factors, stress can lead to changes in the body secretions, especially by the neuroendocrine system, changes in blood circulation, and increased muscle tension. These changes in body chemistry increase susceptibility to physical illness, mental and emotional problems, and accidental injuries.

Stress in its twentieth century variety appears to affect so many disorders not the least of which are anxiety and insomnia. Any herbal remedy, like kava or valerian passiflora, which enhances calmness and relieves anxiety does have a direct connection with our stress levels, and consequently with many major degenerative and autoimmune disorders. It is essential therefore to understand the basis of stress to be able to enhance one's own healing potential.

We used to envy the friendly, relaxed images of islanders from the South Pacific. It now appears that this state was enhanced by drinking kava. Today, via kava products, we have much easier access to the same kavalactones.

Kava will not reorganize your life for you, or remove the stresses; however, in a slightly better mood and with the benefit of a good night's rest, your ability to deal with each stressor and every stressor, combined, may improve.

Sleep Disorders and Fatigue

CHAPTER FIVE

Kava has traditionally been heralded as a sleep-inducing substance.

Almost half the population of industrialized countries will suffer from a diagnosable form of sleep disorder at some time during their lifetime. While this used to be a problem reserved for retirement and old age, so many people in the workforce are "sick and tired of being sick and tired," it almost seems "normal" (at least typical), as everyone else at work is in the same state.

Most companies are operating inefficiently with "half-well" people who are barely getting through each day as it comes. Suburbanites may barely complete the drive home before *crashing* each night and every weekend. We may tell ourselves that all we need is a good night's sleep, yet we endeavor to cope with the pressures of work by using stimulants like coffee, cola drinks, over-the-counter medications, or even black market "uppers." Coffee, donuts and cigarettes may get us through for a while, but are merely stop-gap measures, at best. Then we require more coffee, and stronger than before, together with more donuts and more cigarettes. Soon we gain weight because the donut snack may contribute enough calories to qualify as a whole meal. Meanwhile, our limbs are shaking, and finally we are unable to function mentally, or physically. After getting home from work, we try to rest and relax using hot chocolate, alcohol, black market "downers," etc. Upon retiring to bed, however, we find sleep eludes us. We are unable to get to sleep, or sleep poorly, so that by the next morning we fail to feel properly rested and may have the burden of a hang-over to boot. That proverbial "good night's sleep" becomes ever more elusive. "TGIF" (Thank God It's Friday) is almost a national slogan for the working population!

Sometimes a near wreck on the highway prompts a medical appointment. A number of sleep disorder centers have been established, recently, so more people are seeking an evaluation and medically supervised treatment. More people have become educated to realize that sleep disorders are a serious life-threatening condition and that treatments may be available, if properly diagnosed.

Let's review some of the major sleep disorders and note kava's application to: apnea, insomnia, narcolepsy, periodic limb movements (restless legs) and snoring; as well as some other conditions which may mimic these disorders and be difficult to differentiate, even by a clinician. Most of these other conditions fall under the "umbrella term" of: "Chronic Fatigue Syndrome."

Apnea

Apnea involves, quite simply, an interruption in the breathing rhythm. The person stops breathing for a few seconds, a number of times each night. This may be discerned by a sleep partner, particularly if the person snores (and it is usually quite loud), so that they notice the intervening "sound of silence." It has been estimated that 18 million U.S. citizens suffer from apnea. Most of them don't realize it. Men outnumber women by approximately two to one, in fact four out of every one hundred (4%) men suffer from sleep apnea, but only 2% of women (2 out of every 100).

Most of the time the urge to breathe resumes the respiratory process ... but not always. A number of safety devices have been recommended, while many people receive surgery to correct some abnormality, or restriction, in their airway. However, while surgery (generally involving lasers, these days) usually reduces the snoring, incidents of apnea persist in nearly fifty per cent of patients.

Home treatments for sleep apnea include sleeping on one's side (or being rolled over by a spouse), which can also be helped with simple devices, such as a tennis ball sewn into the neck of a T-shirt, or pajama top. Several taping procedures have been recommended, such as the device worn over the nose by many athletes to improve their breathing. Some sufferers may respond to herbal remedies, including kava, which may provide a deeper sleep, or relax certain muscles.

Insomnia

Insomnia, the most common sleep disorder, is the inability to sleep at all, or the inability to sleep satisfactorily during normal sleeping hours. This condition should only be considered a problem if it impairs daily functioning.

Basic forms of insomnia are: difficulty falling asleep (initial insomnia), difficulty staying asleep, or early morning waking. There may be restless or disturbed sleep, reduction of sleep time (regardless of when the person falls asleep or wakens), and complete wakefulness.

Requirements for sleep vary among individuals and with respect to one individual. For example, children need more sleep than adults. The exact role of sleep and the precise sleep-inducing mechanisms are unknown.

There are many ways to treat insomnia. Some nonmedical treatments include: exercising during the day, going for a walk about an hour before bedtime, reading before bedtime, taking a warm bath, drinking warm milk which contains tryptophan before bed, sexual intercourse, muscle relaxation exercises, meditation and/or, in severe cases, deliberately staying awake for one night to force the resumption of a normal sleep pattern.

The majority of insomnia cases are caused by psychological and emotional problems, such as:

Watching exciting television programs before bedtime
Depression (especially in the case of early morning waking)
Anxiety
Unexpressed anger
Arguing with family members
Fear of dying while sleeping
Virtually any other painful or discomforting disorder.

In Germany, as well as several neighboring European countries, kava preparations are approved for use with cases of insomnia. The action of kava is not fully understood, but one element, aiding the ability to sleep, might be muscular relaxation, which was demonstrated by Meyer in 1962. Other studies, including work by Meyer, again, with animals (mice), have directly associated the administration of kava derivatives (kava pyrones, specifically DHM and DHK) with sleep onset and even sedation. When pigeons were given kava they went into a deep sleep for between two and ten hours! Monkeys fell asleep within fifteen minutes, and remained asleep for over fifteen hours!

Kava may also be useful together with common prescription drugs for insomnia—often barbiturates like sodium pentobarbital (also known as "truth serum"). In such cases, kava has a potentiating action, rendering the other drugs more effective. This could be especially useful in lowering the amount of the prescription drug that is required, possibly even doing away with the addictive components altogether. Kava seems to be non-addictive.

Some manufacturers have combined melatonin with kava, accompanied by claims that kava potentiates (i.e., boosts) the effectiveness of melatonin, which quite independently has compiled an abundant literature testifying to its sleep-enhancing capabilities.

Narcolepsy

Narcolepsy is a sleep disorder in which the sufferer experiences the overwhelming desire to sleep during the day. Attacks may be fleeting, lasting a few seconds, or prolonged, over an hour; in which case they can be disabling for working people.

Basically, the REM (rapid eye movement) of the normal night-time sleep pattern is transferred to the daytime, because it does not occur normally at night. REM usually occurs after one has been asleep for about an hour-and-a-half. In narcoleptics, REM occur upon the onset of sleep. In the U.S., some 50,000 people have been diagnosed with this condition, although estimates are that another 150,000 (200,000 altogether) probably have the disorder but have not brought it to the attention of a physician.

This form of sleep disorder seems to provide a close match with the pattern of sleep induced by kava: deep sleep, with vivid dreaming. REM sleep is the type of sleep during which dreams usually take place.

The ability of kava to induce sound sleep at night, should obviate the need for additional sleep during the day, as well as eliminating attendant symptoms.

Restless Leg Syndrome

Most people have experienced "pins and needles" momentarily when they sit on their legs awkwardly for too long. The syndrome, however, usually strikes at night and combines these sensations with achiness, which is only relieved by movement—walking around the bedroom, for example.

Restless leg syndrome impacts about 15% of the population, to some degree, being most common in middle-aged women.

There is no overt nerve, muscle or circulatory problem associated with Restless Leg Syndrome. There may be rheumatoid arthritis, however, or the patient may be addicted to cigarettes and/or caffeine. The condition is often frequently brought on during pregnancy. It may also be related to hypoglycemia. In one study, one-third of the group experienced both restless legs and spontaneous leg cramps.

Restless legs are usually a symptom of a number of underlying causes. RLS often co-exists with a related sleep disorder called "periodic limb movements in sleep" (PLMS). PLMS features involuntary jerking, or bending, leg movements during sleep every ten to sixty seconds. Some people may experience *hundreds* of such movements per night, which can awaken them, disturb their sleep, and upset their bed partners. It can even lead to divorce!

People who have RLS and PLMS have difficulty both falling asleep as well as staying asleep, and may experience extreme sleepiness during the day (i.e., narcolepsy). This adds difficulties at work, disrupts their social life and may leave them too tired for any recreational activities. As well as "burning the candle" at both ends, working longer to complete their assignments, in an inefficient, soporific state, their quality of work is likely to deteriorate, so that their anxiety or stress levels will soar. They may try to take work home with them, or arrive at work earlier, to make up for it, thereby further compounding the problem.

Although there is no known cause for RLS, in most cases, certain common denominators have been elucidated:

- Family history. RLS runs in some families.
- Pregnancy. Some women experience RLS during pregnancy, especially in the third trimester, recovering following delivery.
- Low iron levels (anemia). For these patients, iron supplements correct both the anemia and RLS symptoms.
- Chronic diseases. Diabetes, kidney failure, peripheral neuropathy and rheumatoid arthritis may be associated with RLS.
- Caffeine intake. Decreasing caffeine intake may relieve symptoms.

Kava has been reported to be beneficial in relieving RLS. Presumably, it works by inducing a state of muscular relaxation which facilitates sleep. Of course, this initiates a positive, rather than a vicious cycle, so that because of the restful sleep, muscles are better able to relax.

Chronic Fatigue Syndrome

Chronic Fatigue Syndrome is an all-encompassing term for symptoms which may actually result from the same or similar source. There is currently some debate whether there are several names for the same disease, or different stages of one disease, or separate diseases with similar symptoms:

- Autoimmune disorder
- Candida Albicans
- Chronic mononucleosis
- Cytomegalovirus
- Epstein-Barr virus
- Herpes simplex virus
- Myalgic encephalomyelitis (ME)
- Yuppie 'flu

Patients suffering from any of these syndromes may be fatigued and suffer chronic symptoms of a mild infection. The favorite theory of causation is that of a viral infection. Which virus, is another matter. There certainly appears to be a continuum of herpes virus, mononucleosis and Epstein-Barr. However, such conditions need not assert themselves if the host is not compromised, whether with a toxic bowel, or depressed immune system, or both. Hence, natural treatments for these diseases tend to aim at detoxification and immune support.

Some other common Chronic Fatigue symptoms, often presenting together, include:

- Headache
- Intestinal discomfort
- Low-grade fever
- Lymph node swelling
- Muscle and joint pain
- Recurrent sore throat

Overall, two key symptoms recur in most of these disorders: muscle tension and sleep deprivation. In the search for a "cure," or at least a treatment, what product achieves these two objectives: providing muscular relaxation and sleep? As we have discussed, kava seems to be a perfect match! The appropriateness of kava still needs to be considered relative to an accurate evaluation of the person's real needs. Kava may also enhance restful sleep and its associated dreams. It may even mask the discomfort of a headache, joint pain, or sore throat. It may have other benefits as well, but it is better to reserve judgment until the evidence accumulates further before regarding kava as a universal panacea.

For the moment, anyway, recommending kava as a "cure" for Chronic Fatigue, as an example, seems to be a gross over-statement. In the first place, we are not even sure what precisely Chronic Fatigue is. Prescribing from a diagnostic label is not the (w)holistic approach, anyway. The approach is more along the lines of: is the person under stress, sleeping poorly, with a compromised immune system and chronic ill health? You don't opt for kava because of the particular illness. You seek to resolve the root of the problem, by removing certain stressors and facilitating relaxation and proper rest. This is an appropriate use of kava, either by itself or in conjunction with other herbs, or nutrients.

Cynics can continue to carp that the benefits of kava are "unproven." Certainly, even if kava does not overcome the viral foundation of so-called Chronic Fatigue, the fact that the patients feel and sleep better may boost their immune system sufficiently to effect an improvement. The virus may not have been eradicated, but may stay in remission as long as the host's immune system is functioning properly.

Kava, then, may not be a cure, or even bring about a cure by and of itself. It may set the stage, however. That in itself may be all that is required; thereby making kava a sound investment. [More details concerning the pharmacology of kava are contained in Chapter 2. The Scientific Evidence So Far.]

Other Uses

Traditionally, kava was sometimes considered to be too potent for the sick or infirm. Generally, however, it has always been classified as a medicinal plant as well as a ceremonial beverage. Kilham reports that the primary folk-medicinal use was for urogenital inflammation and cystitis. Kava first appeared in the U.S. Dispensatory for urinary tract infections (UTI's) and by 1950 was found in two medicinal preparations: *Gonosan* for gonorrhea and *Neurocardin* for nervous disorders. Together with other reports, the following picture can be built up:

Abortifacient
Tradition dictated that most women avoid drinking kava. In some societies it would have been considered a major taboo because of the origin stories, in which kava grew from a woman's body. There may be some substance to the fact that kava may have been

associated with sterility.   It is claimed to be able to induce a miscarriage.

Anesthetic

Simply chewing (mastication) kava root numbs (anesthetizes) the mouth. Meyer identified the specific kavalactone responsible for this effect, which turned out to be kavain. He recommended their use as superficial anesthetics because they are free of toxicity. Baldi has cautioned against too high a dose, which can paralyze peripheral nerves.

There is an obvious similarity to the effect of cocaine, which provides a number of topical and injectable solutions, marketed as: *Lidocaine*, *Marcaine* and *Novocaine*.

Analgesic

Kava's two most powerful lactones: DHK and DHM have been compared with common analgesics, including: aspirin and morphine. Morphine is, of course, the most potent, requiring a mere 2.5 mgs per kilogram, but DHK and DHM were equal at 120 mgs, half the dosage required for aspirin (acetylsalicyclic acid).

Contraceptive

Following childbirth, new mothers took the tea to stop from becoming pregnant again too soon. At other times chewing the leaves was deemed to provide contraceptive benefits.   It is also likely that it would relieve any lingering pain and promote sleep.

Diuretic action

In Fiji the root tea was used in cases of kidney and bladder ailments because of its diuretic action. It was also used for coughs, colds and sore throats, undoubtedly due to its numbing action (not unlike the popular throat lozenge *Chloraseptic*).

Epilepsy

Pfeiffer reported some initial trials with kava extracts as anticonvulsant agents in persons with epilepsy (1967). While there was some improvement in seizure control, the trial was stopped owing to subtle skin changes.

It may be that as our pharmacological understanding of kava improves, we may be able to isolate the anticonvulsant agent as well as the dermopathogen and, thereby, solve both problems at the same time!

Fungal infections

The kava bars (*nakamals*) of Vanuatu are able to prepare kava several days in advance, leaving it exposed to the elements. Therefore, it seems resistant to spoilage.

Opinions differ whether kava has a bactericidal effect. Steinmetz did confirm that it did possess such a property with respect to gonococus (gonorrhea) as well as colon bacillus, and others have added Salmonella typhi.

Hansel has been particularly impressed with kava's efficacy against mycoses (fungal infections) of the skin, which has proven to be very resistant to treatment generally. Indeed, a common medication, *griseofulvine*, has no effect on Aspergillus niger, which is completely inhibited by DHK (dihydrokavain).

Duve has proposed taking this one step further and utilizing kavalactones as natural preservatives in foods.

Menopause

Warnecke undertook a study (1991) with a group of menopausal women suffering from problems with muscular control (dystonia). The measured variable was an anxiety scale, which revealed an improvement in the kava group after the very first week! Other improvements were also noted, which may be even more important, including an overall improvement in their general mood and sense of well being, as well as a reduction in common symptoms, like hot flashes. No side effects were reported.

Thermogenic

Uses for the leaves are also mentioned in some sources, including a leaf poultice for headaches. Traditionally, feverish patients were given a bed of leaves to help them perspire (sudorific), to break a cold or fever. Similarly, kava is also thought to be "thermogenic," which means that it can raise the heat of the body's thermostat so that it burns more fuel. In this manner, it has been traditionally used to bring people back to normal weight and fitness.

The first pharmaceutical preparations were also German, dating from the 1920s. The kava tincture was sold as a mild sedative and hypotensive (for lowering blood pressure, the condition of high blood pressure being termed: hypertension).

By 1914 kava was listed in the British Pharmacopeia and was firmly established as a sedative and hypotensive throughout Europe shortly after the First World War in the "Roaring 1920s."

Treating Wounds
Juice from the leaves was also used to treat open wounds. Once again, the numbing function may have been the key. Kava, in some form, has also been found to be useful for other minor skin problems, including bites, stings and fungal infections.

Venereal diseases
A twenty percent oil of kava resin in oil of sandalwood, called *Gonosan*, has been used internally for gonorrhea.

Norton regards the use for gonorrhea as a thing of the past, at least in Europe. It is a strange quirk of fate that, by many estimations, while the Polynesians gave the British navy the gift of kava, venereal disease may have been what they got in return!

On the lighter side, the free love in the South Seas was too good to be true for the British sailors under Cook and other explorers. Hence they would provide their girlfriends with a token of their appreciation. The most popular item became the ship's nails. Once the ship's stores ran out of their supply, sailors began pulling nails from the ship itself, causing Cook to order a stop to the practice, for fear that his ship would fall apart!

In Japan, kava was in use against gonorrhea prior to the Second World War. Kava had been used prophylactically by the islanders and Japanese settlers had reported the benefits back to Japan. A mechanism has never been substantiated and the developments in antibiotics following the war made kava redundant.

Contemporary Medicinal Uses

Today, European herbal and pharmaceutical manufacturers annually require one hundred tons of kava for a wide range of products, mostly in combination with other ingredients. Just to cite a few examples from each country:

- **England**: *Antiglan* and *Protat* for bladder discomfort; and "GB tablets" for the gall bladder.
- **France**: *Kaviase* for urinary tract infections.
- **Germany**: *Arthrosetten* for arthritis; *Cysto Fink* for urinary tract infections; *Hewepsychon* for psychiatric disorders; *Kavain Harras* for restlessness, stress and psychosomatic conditions; *Kavasporal* (which comes in a pure form as well as combination compounds) and *Laitan* (which only comes in a pure form) which are both used for anxiety and nervous disorders; *Somnuvis* which is for nervousness; and *Valeriana* which is for sleeplessness and nervousness.

- **Switzerland**: *Cysto-Caps* for bladder problems; and *Kawaform* which is a general tonic.

The British Herbal Pharmacopoeia recognizes kava as: antimicrobial, diuretic, spasmolytic, sedative, carminative (removing bloating and flatulence) and as a topical rubefacient, for use in the treatment of cystitis, urethritis, rheumatism, joint pains (topical); specific indication is infection of genitourinary tract. Combined with marshmallow, celery seed and couchgrass in bladder disease; with buck bean, black cohosh and celery seed in rheumatism. A standard homeopathic *Materia Medica* lists the use of kava for headache and neurasthenia.

Lebot's List
Lebot, co-author of *Kava, the Pacific Drug*, even included a table in which the specific form of kava used in treatments was given. At the present time, most of these can only be replicated in the South Seas, owing to the availability of whole, fresh, kava plants.

Condition	Folk Medical Treatment
Abortifacient	Kava leaves intra-vaginally
Anesthetic	Masticated kava root
Asthma	Macerated stump drink
Chest (Pulmonary) pain	Masticated kava drink
Chills	Macerated kava drink, or fumigation with leaves

Chills & insomnia	Masticated, macerated kava diluted with water & boiled
Conjunctivitis	Eyewash of diluted leaf juice
Constipation	Kava drink
Contraception	Masticating and swallowing kava leaves
Cuts	Kava leaf juice
Cystitis	Kava drink
Diaphoresis	Kava drink
Diarrhea	Kava drinks
Difficulties urinating	Macerated stump drink
Dysmenorrhea	Kava drink
Edema	Bathing & applying poultices of kava leaves
Fever	Drink made from kava leaves
Gastrointestinal upsets	Macerated stump drink with other medicinal plants
General treatment of disease	Fumigation with leaves
General weakness (Fatigue)	Masticated, macerated kava diluted with water & boiled
Gonorrhea	Kava drink
Headaches (1)	Infusion of masticated kava root tissues
Headaches (2)	Hot leaves are placed on the head
Immune builder	Masticated kava drink
Labor	Juice from kava leaves
Leprosy	External application of masticated stump
Menarche	Masticated kava drink
Migraine (female)	Masticated kava drink

Rheumatism	Macerated stump drink
Sedative	Drink from scraped & pounded kava root
Skin diseases	Poultice of masticated stump
Sore throat	Scraped bark and masticated roots
Suppuration	Poultice of masticated stump
Tonic	Kava leaf juice
Toothache	Internal part of kava bark
Urogenital inflammation	Drink of macerated stump and young kava shoots
Weight gain	Macerated stump drink

Some of these uses may never be verified, scientifically, since they reflect the symbolism of the plant within the prevailing culture and, perhaps, even attendant beliefs, including illnesses brought on by sorcery as a result of a broken taboo. So, just as a life-giving fluid flows forth from the kava roots, kava was deemed to promote lactation.

Dosages and Specific Applications

To gain some perspective on the parameters of kava intake, whether for recreation, or therapeutic purposes, a review of various dosages is in order.

The standard half-cup of kava drink contains approximately 250 milligrams of kavalactones, which is more than enough to assist the average person in going to sleep, although social gatherings would involve several (five or more) servings, even though there is no necessity for it, so far as sleep, or health, are concerned.

Research studies have used varying quantities and concentrations. The 70% concentration is usually taken three times a day (t.i.d.) in dosages of either 100 or 200 milligrams (mgs), between 300 and 600 mgs per day. Comparing the kavalactone concentration, the clinical, or therapeutic, dose of 300 mg at 70% concentration is equivalent to 210 mg of kavalactones. Therefore, this daily dose is about the same as one shell of the traditional beverage. The recommendation to take this strength of kava, in one dose, at night for sleep is also well within traditional consumption levels.

Most over-the-counter kava preparations sold in the U.S. have a lower concentration, 30%. The abuse in Australia may have involved 4 grams (4,000 milligrams) of kavalactones. (This would equate to 30 capsules; or in liquid form, 1 ml is equivalent to 250 mg.) Even at this level, the only problem known to be attributable to kava was the dermopathy. The researchers identified a threshold level of more than 310 grams per week before encountering problems. In round numbers, this is 1,000 times the daily therapeutic dose. No confirmed cases of kava dermopathy have been recorded while taking recommended levels of standardized kava extracts.

Dermopathy

Georg Foster, Captain Cook's botanist, who also named the kava plant, recorded the associated dermopathy thus: "Cutis exarescere et in squamulas exfoliari." (The skin dries up and exfoliates in little scales.)

In spite of this recognition of an association between kava drinking and a skin condition (called *kani* in Fiji) within traditional societies, upon first sight the current literature reveals only three studies, between 1958 and 1994, which attempt to understand the underlying pharmacological basis for this skin condition and the possible therapeutic approaches.

The problem does appear to be reversible, if kava drinking is reduced, or refrained from completely, so long as a balanced diet was available. (We have already noted that in some traditional societies, kava drinkers wore their scales as a "badge of honor"! This was noted early on, by Cook's lieutenant, James King, who wrote: "The skin begins to be covered with a whitish scurf, like the leprosy, which many regard as a badge of nobility....")

The skin becomes very dry and scaly, somewhat fish-like, hence its official na...e: ichthyosiform eruption. In the common vernacular today, we might refer to "lizard legs." The shins are a prime area, as well as the palms of the hands, the soles of the feet, the forearms and back. A report from a merchant seaman records the progression of the condition as follows: head, face, neck and body. This progression was observed both in where the scales first broke out, as well as the order in which they cleared up. This sounds a little like part of the credo of homeopathy, hence it is no surprise that kava should be tried as a cure for pre-existing skin conditions, first exacerbating matters and then as the scales cleared, taking with them the pre-existing disorder, leaving (it is claimed) a clear skin underneath.

While Polynesian legends regard the skin affliction as a reminder of an ancient legend, or even a curse, modern science continues to be at a loss, other than a wide range of speculation, including:
• accumulated plant pigments
• chronic allergic dermatitis

- interference with glandular secretions
- pellagra (i.e. niacin deficiency)
- photo-sensitivity.

The first study, conducted by Frater in Fiji, proposed that kava disrupted some unknown mechanism of B-vitamin metabolism, in the same manner as pellagra. The follow-up study did not take place until much later (1990) when Ruze gathered some Tongan kava drinkers, all with the dermopathy, who were divided into two groups. One group received a niacin supplement. The control group received a placebo (an inert substance, usually sugar, providing no nutritional benefit other than a few *empty* calories). Surprisingly, about one-third of each group showed signs of improvement! A niacin deficiency does not seem, therefore, to be the metabolic pathway.

Ruze suggested that kava interferes with cholesterol metabolism, parallel to lipid-lowering agents such as triparanol. Ruze, together with the first-named author, Norton, most recently (1994) concluded that the kava products sold by the health food industry retain the inherent risk of leading to kava disorders. However, they recognize that a "health-food enthusiast would need to consume an enormous quantity of kava to affect the skin, so it is unlikely that kava dermopathy will occur in temperate users."

Safety and Toxicity

As we noted earlier, circumstances are such that controlled trials of kava will probably not be undertaken. Each of us is an experiment of one! So, if you have a problem which sounds like it may be helped by kava, you can make an informed decision on your own behalf. Always try a small dose of something first and then give the recommended dose a try for a week or two in order to judge its efficacy.

Typical kava use is three times daily, although this may vary with the purpose, the patient and the form of kava being used. The following guidelines appear in the literature:

Dosages

The dosage used will depend upon the level of kavalactones in a preparation.

For anxiety-relieving effects: Capsules contain between 45 - 70 mg of kava Standardized for kavalactones, and can be taken 3 - 4 times a day.

For sedative effects: One may take up to 210 mg two hours before bedtime.

Kava is also being combined with other herbs in a number of herbal products being marketed, today. A natural aid to mental well being is touted as being a mixture of kava with St. John's Wort (Hypericum).

Additional Chinese herbs may be added, such as: Bupleurum, Dong Quai, Licorice and Peony.

To enhance sleep, the following mixture is being recommended: Melatonin - 3 mg., Kava Root Extract - 250 mg., B-6 - 10 mg.

Drug Comparison

Munte compared the effects of oxazepam and an extract of kava roots on event-related potentials in a word recognition task. The subjects' task was to identify, within a list of visually presented words, those that were shown for the first time and those that were being repeated. Oxazepam led to a significantly worse recognition rate. Kava subjects, on the other hand, showed a slightly increased recognition rate and a larger ERP difference between old and new words.

Munte, T.F., et al. "Effects of oxazepam and an extract of kava roots (Piper methysticum) on event-related potentials in a word recognition task." *Neuropsychobiology.* 1993; 27(1): 46-53.

Contraindications

The U.S. FDA has determined kava kava resin acts on the spinal column. Kava may produce unknown damage to the liver. Further, it is recommended that one avoids driving while under the influence of kava.

The monograph prepared by the German regulatory body (which is likely to be the gold standard throughout the world now that it is available in English) regards kava use as potentially harmful during pregnancy and lactation, which has been echoed on some product lines in the U.S.. It is also stated to be contraindicated in cases of deep depression.

Drug Interactions

Known Interactions

Insofar as diuretic action, kava kava increases the renal excretion of sodium and chloride, which may potentiate the hyperglycemic and hyperuremic effects of glucose elevating agents.

Possible Interactions

Kava kava's analgesic effects may be additive with other analgesics and anesthetics. It may be inhibited by barbiturates even though CNS depressant effects may occur.

The analgesic property of this herb may be reversed or eliminated by p-chlorophenylalanine, cyproheptadine HCl, and phenobarbital.

The CNS depressant tendency of this analgesic may be potentiated by chlorpoxthixene HCl, haloperidol, and tranquilizers.

The antacid nature of kava kava may decrease or delay the absorption of nalidixic acid and the sulfon-amides.

Due to the spasmolytic nature of kava kava it may interact in unknown ways with CNS depressants or stimulants.

The use of diuretics may require dosage adjustments of antidiabetic drugs.

Kava kava should not be used with metho-trimeprazine, a potent CNS depressant analgesic.

Comments

In the absence of other hard data, it may still be assumed that observable interactions may occur between the many central nervous system drugs and the psychoactive principles in this herb.

Kava does not appear to be a narcotic, though opinion is divided on this point. Continued use may cause inflammation of body and eyes, resulting ulcers, parching and peeling of skin. But, high doses of kava are unnecessary, and should not be encouraged by health care providers.

. Judging whether any untoward side effects are due to a reaction to kava, or are, simply, proof that kava is benefiting you, helping rid your body of toxins, may pose a problem. In a number of naturopathic proto-cols, including homeopathy, some symptoms are to be expected, if the treatment is working. This can include a "healing crisis" with a fever, or a gastro-intestinal disruption, encompassing vomiting and/or diarrhea.

If you purchase kava products at the health store and make the decision to use them on your own, you may still seek a consultation with a naturopathic provider, who may be familiar with anticipated effects.

Another ruse that is often perpetrated by opponents of health food stores is the lack of standardization of the products. Standardization poses a problem in many cases. Indeed, if the products are imported whole, processing of some type may be required to satisfy the shipping and customs authorities so that no harmful pests are brought in as well. Certainly, purists would abhor radiation of the product, or pesticide usage. However, importers may have little choice in the matter. Other logistical concerns include the time it takes for the shipments to reach the market. Most native consumers are not faced with these issues, as they cut their own fresh roots.

Mechanization is making inroads, even in the South Seas, so that urban dwellers, in particular, on larger islands may prefer the convenience of a powder from their nearby store to the more traditional root.

Some of these larger suppliers are tackling the import market directly, which should help their credibility. These may be found on the Internet. Virtually the full range of products is now being offered at specialty stores and through mail order (or 'Net order??), from roots, to chips, to powders and capsules on to extracts and tinctures. The only glaring omission is sale of the leaves, which is an impracticality.

Moreover, there have been concerns about impurities, or adulteration. Once the parts are ground into a

powder, it is difficult to tell, visually, what the concentration of lactones may be. However, chemical testing
can be introduced to overcome this problem. Be sure to
always obtain your kava from a reputable supplier of
herbs.

Abstracts

Some specific studies address issues of: alcohol and dermopathy.

Alcohol

One obvious question with a recreational mood enhancer is how it will react if taken with alcohol. Herberg studied safety-related performance when kava was administered together with ethyl alcohol (0.05% blood alcohol concentration).

The results showed no negative multiplicative effects caused by the kava-special extract. With the concentration test, however, there was a remarkable advantage of the extract group. This supports previous work with native drinkers, undertaken by Singh. Kava had no effect on their reaction times or errors.

Herberg, K.W. "Effect of Kava-Special Extract WS 1490 combined with ethyl alcohol on safety-relevant performance parameters." *Blutalkohol.* 1993 Mar; 30(2): 96-105.

Anxiety

This fairly long trial, also used WS 1490 and the duration proved significant, as benefits did not reach significance until week 8. With continued use, other benefits became apparent, notably the excellent side-effect profile, which omitted the usual dependency associated with anti-depressant medication.

This trial used the same dosage that had been established in short-term trials, i.e., 90 - 110 mg dry extract t.i.d. (three times a day) equivalent to 70 mg kavalactones, each time.

Kava is rated as being a promising possibility to treat anxiety disorders.

Volz, H.P. "Kava kava extract WS 1490 versus placebo in anxiety disorder—a randomized, placebo-controlled 25 week outpatient trial." *Pharmacopsyc.* 1997, 30: 1-5.

Reports like this have supported the use of kava in Germany, where it is classified as a tranquilizer and accounts for $8 million worth of herbal sales.

Kava Dermopathy: Allergic skin reactions

Suss and Lehmann address a common concern, that of allergic skin reactions to kava root extract. They cite the well known side effect (ichthyosiform kava dermopathy, i.e., scaly skin like a fish) of excessive use of kava and provide a case report of an acute allergic side effect to kava extract.

Suss, R. and Lehmann, P. "Hematogenous contact eczema cause by phytogenic drugs exemplified by kava root extract." *Hautarzt*. 1996 Jun; 47(6): 459-61.

Norton and Ruze regard the problem as reversible. This topic is covered at greater length in Chapter 6.

Norton, S.A. and Ruze, P. "Kava dermopathy." *J-Am-Acad-Dermatol*. 1994 Jul; 31(1): 89-97.

Frequently Asked Questions

If you have read the book diligently, you have acquired an in-depth knowledge about kava. If you are scanning through for answers to key questions, you may like to review this summary.

What should I look for in a quality kava product?

While premium raw products may have greater potency, especially when freshly harvested, the general consensus is to opt for a standardized extract. Go by the amount of kavalactones, rather than the overall weight of the capsule. (The standard half-cup of kava drink contains approximately 250 milligrams of kavalactones, which is more than enough to assist the average person in going to sleep.) The kavalactone content should be stated clearly on the product. Of course, some of these statements can be incorrect, although reputable companies will test their raw materials and processes more thoroughly.

Is kava better in the capsule form than a liquid?

Traditionally, the root was processed and made into a beverage. Modern processing and consumer preferences dictate that the root is powdered. This can then be encapsulated, directly, or subjected to further processing to provide a modern equivalent of the beverage or a tincture. The tincture can be unpleasant for some people to take, so capsules are probably the most popular form. However, as with many other products, some people feel that they absorb the liquid product better than the capsule. Yet, if the kavalactone concentration is proportionate, the effect should be the same. It comes down to individual preferences.

If I take kava during the day, will it cause sleepiness?

Kava has an established reputation as an evening drink resulting in deep sleep, without a hangover. However, ceremonials usually took place during the day. It is a matter of dosage. To combat anxiety, for example, three doses of kava are recommended during the day. To promote sleep, a single amount, equal to three therapeutic doses (or one traditional beverage), is common practice.

Indeed, a small amount of kava seems to intensify perceptions of sound and vision, rather than having a sedative effect.

Above all, people report an enhanced mood and a state of calmness which is difficult to achieve otherwise in our hectic modern world.

Bibliography

Abbott, I.A., and C. Shimazu. "The geographic origin of the plants most commonly used for medicine by Hawaiians." *Journal of Ethnopharmacology.* 14, nos. 2 & 3 (1985): 213-222.

American Herbal Products Association. *Kava Symposium Proceedings.* 1997. Bethesda, Maryland. (In Press.)

Anonymous. "Kava." *Lancet.* 1988 Jul 30; 2 (8605): 258-9.

Anonymous. "Kava-kava: a calming herb from the South Pacific." *Herbs for Health.* January/February, 1997: 42-44.

Backhauss, L. and Kriegistein, J. "Extract of kava (Piper methysticum) and its methysticum constituents protect brain tissue against ischemic damage in rodents." *Eur J Pharmacol.* 215 (1992): 265-269.

Baldi, D. "Sulle proprieta farmacologische del Piper methysticum." *Terapia moderna.* 1980, 4: 359-64.

Bibra, Baron Ernst von. *Plant Intoxicants.* Rochester, Vt.: Healing Arts Press, 1995.

Biersack, A. "Kava onau and the Tongan chiefs." *Journal of the Polynesian Society.* 100 (1991): 231-268.

Borsche, W. and Lewinsohn, M. "Untersuchungen uber die Bestandteile der Kawawurzel, 1: Uber Yangonin." *Cheische Berichte.* 1933, 66: 1792-1801.

Bott, E. "Kava ceremony in Tonga: Psychoanalysis and ceremony." In: *The Interpretation of Ritual.* ed. J.S. La Fontaine. London: Tavistock, 1972.

Brenneis, D. "Grog and gossip in Bhatgaon: Style and substance in Fiji Indian conversation." *American Ethnologist.* 11 (1984): 487-506.

British Herbal Medicine Association. *British Herbal Pharmacopoeia.* 1983.

Brunton, R. "A harmless substance? Anthropological aspects of kava in the South Pacific." In: Prescott, J. and McCall, G. eds. "Kava: use and abuse in Australia and the South Pacific." National Drug and Alcohol Research Centre, Sydney, University of NSW *Monograph No. 5.* 1989: 13 - 25.

Brunton, R. *The Abandoned Narcotic. Kava and Cultural Instability in Melanesia.* Cambridge, England: Cambridge University Press, 1989.

Buckley, J.P., et al. "Pharmacology of kava." In: *Ethnopharmacologic Search for Psychoactive Drugs.* D.H. Efron et al, eds. Public Health Service, Pbn no. 1645. Washington, D.C.: U.S. GPO. 1967.

Cambie, R.C. and Ash, J. *Fijian Medicinal Plants.* Australia. CSIRO. 1994.

Capasso, A. and Pinto, A. "Experimental investigations of the synergistic-sedative effect of passiflora and kava." *Acta Therapeutica.* 21 (2) (1995): 127-140.

Cawte, J. "Psychoactive substances of the South Seas: Betel, kava and pituri." *Australia and New Zealand Journal of Psychiatry.* 1985; 19 (1): 83-7.

Cawte, J. "Parameters of kava used as a challenge to alcohol." *Aus. & N.Z. J. Psychiatry.* 1986(20): 70-76.

Cheng, D. et al. "Identification of methane chemical ionization gas chromatography/mass spectroscopy of the products obtained by steam distillation and aqueous extraction of commercial Piper Meth." *Biomed. Env. Mass. Spectroscopy.* 1988, 17(5): 371-376.

Chew, W.L. "The genus Piper (Piperaceae) in New Guinea, Solomon Islands and Australia." *Journal of the Arnold Arboretum.* 53 (1972): 1-25.

Chinnery, E.W.P. "Piper methysticum in betel chewing." *Man.* 22 (1922): 24-27.

Cowling, W. "Kava and tradition in Tonga ," In: *Kava use and abuse in Australia and the South Pacific,* ed. Prescott, J. and McCall, G. Monograph no. 5. Sydney, Australia: University of New South Wales, National Drug and Alcohol Research Centre, 1988.

Cox, P.A., and Banack, S.A. eds. *Islands, Plants, and Polynesians: An Introduction to Polynesian Ethnobotany.* Portland, OR: Dioscorides Press, 1991.

Cox, P.A., and O'Rourke, L. "Kava (Piper methysticum, Piperaceae)." *Economic Botany.* 41, no. 3 (1987): 452-454.

Cox, P.A., et al. "Pharmacological Activity of the Samoan ethnopharmacopoeia." *Economic Botany.* 43, no. 4 (1989): 487-497.

Cuzent, G. "Rapport sur la composition chimique de la kavahine." *Cahiers de l'Academie des Sciences.* 1861, 52: 205-6.

D'Abbs, P. "The power of kava or the power of ideas? Kava use and kava policy in the Northern Territory, Australia." Paper presented at the 17th Pacific Science Congress, Honolulu, Hawaii, 1991.

Davies, L P. et al. "Kava pyrones and resin: studies on GABAA, GABAB, and benzodiazepine binding sites in rodent brain." *Pharmacology and Toxicology.* 71 (1992): 120-126.

Du Toit, B.M. *Drugs, rituals and altered states of consciousness.* Rotterdam: A.A. Balkema, 1977.

Duffield, A.M., Lidgard, R.O. and Low, G.K. "Analysis of the constituents of Piper methysticum by gas chromatography methane chemical ionization mass spectrometry: New trace constituents of kava resin." *Biomedical and Environmental Mass Spectrometry.* 13 (1986): 305-313.

Duffield, P.H. and Jamieson, D. "Development of tolerance to kava in mice." *Clin Exp Pharmacol Physiol.* 18 (1991): 571-578.

Duke, J.A. *CRC Handbook of Medicinal Herbs.* CRC Press, Inc., Boca Raton, Florida, 1985.

Dutta, C.P. et al. "Studies on the genus of Piper." *Journal of the Indian Chemistry Society.* 1976. 55.

Dutta, C.P. "Constituents of flavokawain-C.Pipermethysticum." *Indian Journal of Chemistry* 11 (1973): 509-5 10.

Duve, R.N. "Highlight of the chemistry and pharmacology of yaqona, Piper methysticum." *Fiji Agricultural Journal.* 38 (1976): 81-84.

Duve, R.N. "Gas-liquid chromatographic determination of major constituents of Piper methysticum." *Analyst.* 106 (1981): 160-165.

Duve, R.N. "Quality evaluation of yaqona (Piper methysticum) in Fiji." *Fiji Agricultural Journal.* 43 (1981): 1-8.

Duve, R.N. and Prasad, V. "Changes in chemical composition of Yaqona (Piper methysticum) with time." *Fiji Agricultural Journal.* 45 (1983): 45-60.

Duve, R.N. and Prasad, V. "Efficacy of extraction of constituents in the preparation of yaqona beverage. Part 1: General constituents." *Fiji Agricultural Journal.* 1984 (46): 5 - 9.

Duve, R.N. and Prasad, V. "Efficacy of extraction of constituents in the preparation of yaqona beverage. Part 2: General constituents." *Fiji Agric. J.* 1984 (46): 11 - 16.

Efron, D.H. et al. eds. *Ethnopharmacologic Search for Psychoactive Drugs.* Public Health Service, Pbn no. 1645. Washington, D.C.: U.S. GPO. 1967.

Ellis, R.W. "Kava benefits Australian aborigines." *Pacific Islands Monthly*. 55 (1984): 27-28.

Feldman, H. "Informal kava drinking in Tonga." *Journal of the Polynesian Society*. 89 (1980): 101-103.

Finau, S.A., Stanhope, J.M. and Prior, I.A.M.. "Kava, alcohol and tobacco consumption among Tongas with urbanization." *Social Science and Medicine*. 16 (1982): 35-41.

Ford, C.S. "Ethnographical aspects of kava." In: *EthnopharmacologicSearch for Psychoactive Drugs*, ed. Efron, D.H. et al.

Foster, S. "Kava-kava: A gift of calm from the South pacific." *Better Nutrition*. May, 1997. 54-59.

Frater, A.S. "Medical aspects of yaqona." *Transactions and Proceedings of the Fijian Society*. 5 (1952): 31-39.

Freund, P. and Marshall, M. "Research bibliography of alcohol and kava studies in oceania: update and additional items." *Micronesia*. 1977(13): 313-317.

Furgiule, A.R., Kinnard, W.J., Aceto, M.D. and Buckley, J.P. "Central activity of aqueous extracts of Piper methysticum (kava)." *Journal of Pharmaceutical Sciences*. 154 (1965): 247-252.

Gajdusek, D.C. "Recent observations on the use of kava in the New Hebrides." In: *Ethnopharmacologic Search for Psychoactive Drugs*. ed. Efron, D.H. et al. Public Health Service Publication no. 1645. Washington, D.C.: U.S. Government Printing Office, 1967, 119-125.

Garner, L. F., and Klinger, J.D. "Some visual effects caused by the beverage kava." *Journal of Ethnopharmacology*. 13, no. 3 (1985): 307-311.

Gatty, R. "Kava: Polynesian beverage shrub." *Economic Botany*. 10 (1956): 241-249.

Gaus, W. and Hogel, J. "Studies on the efficacy of unconventional therapies. Problems and designs." *Arzneimittelforschung*. 1995 Jan; 45(1): 88-92.

German Commission Extract Monographs, *Kava-kava rhizome*. 1990. Translated by American Botanical Council. (1997.)

Gleitz, J. et al. "(+/-)-Kavain inhibits veratridine-activated voltage-dependent Na(+)-channels in synaptosomes prepared from rat cerebral cortex." *Neuropharmacology*. 1995 Sep; 34(9): 1133-8.

Gobley, M. "Recherches chimiques sur la racine de kava." *J. de Pharmacie et de Chimie*. 1860, 37:19-23.

Gregory, R.J., Gregory, J.E. and Peck, J.G.. "Kava and prohibition in Tanna, Vanuatu." *British Journal of Addiction.* 76 (1981): 299-313.

Hansel, R. et al. "Fungistatic effect of kava." *Archiv der Pharmazie.* 229 (1966): 507-512.

Hansel, R. and Beiersdorf, H.U. "Zur kenttnis der sedativen prinzipien des Kava-rhizoms." *Arz. Forsch.* 1959, 9:581-5.

Heinze, H.J. et al. "Pharmacopsychological effects of oxazepam and kava-extract in a visual search paradigm assessed with event-related potentials." *Pharmacopsychiatry.* 1994 Nov; 27(6): 224-30.

Herb Research Foundation. "The safety of Piper Methysticum." Report. Presented at the 1997 Kava Symposium. [Published by Singh and Blumenthal.]

Herberg, K.W. "Effect of Kava-Special Extract WS 1490 combined with ethyl alcohol on safety-relevant performance parameters." *Blutalkohol.* 1993 Mar; 30(2): 96-105.

Hoffer, A. and Osmond, H. *The Hallucinogens.* With a contribution by T. Weckowicz, "Animal studies of hallucinogenic drugs." New York: Academic Press, 1967.

Hocart, C.H., et al. "Chemical archaeology of kava, a potent brew." *Rapid Commun. Mass-Spectrom.* 1993 Mar; 7(3): 219-24.

Holm, E., et al. "Studies on the profile of the neurophysiological effects of D,L - kavain: Cerebral sites of action and sleep-wakefulness-rhythm in animals." *Arzneimittel-Forsch.* 41 (1991): 673-683.

Holmes, L.D. "The function of kava in modern Samoan culture." In: *Ethnopharmacologic Search for Psychoactive Drugs.* ed. D.H. Efron, et al.

Holmes, L.D. "The Samoan kava ceremony: Its forms and functions." *Science of Man.* 1, (1961): 46-5 1.

Hough, W. "Kava drinking as practiced by the Papuans and Polynesians." Smithsonian Institution Miscellaneous Collection 47 (1904): 85-92.

Jamieson, D.D., et al. "Comparison of the central nervous system activity of the aqueous and lipid extracts of kava (Piper Methysticum)." *Arch. Int. de Pharm. et de Ther.* 301 (1989): 66 - 80.

Jamieson, D.D. and Duffield, P.H. "The antinociceptive action of kava components in mice." *Clin. Exp. Pharmacol. Physiol.* 17 (1990): 495-508.

Jose, J. and Sharma, A.K. "Structure and behaviour of chromosomes in Piper and Peperomia (family Piperaceae)." *Cytologia.* 50 (1985): 301-310.

Jossang, P. and Molho, D.. "Dihydrokavain has sedative properties like dihydromethysticin." *Journal of Chromatography.* 31 (1970): 375.

Jussogie, A. et al. "Kavapyrone extract enriched from Piper methysticum as modulator of the GABA binding site in different regions of rat brain." *Psychopharmacology-Berl.* 1994 Dec; 116(4): 469-74.

Keledjian, J., et al. "Uptake into mouse brain of four compounds present in the psychoactive beverage kava." *Journal of Pharmaceutical Sciences.* 77 (1988): 1,003-1,006.

Keller, F. and Klohs, M.W. "A review of the chemistry and pharmacology of the constituents of Piper methysticum." *Lloydia.* 26 (1963): 1-15.

Kilham, C. *Kava: Medicine Hunting in Paradise: the pursuit of a Natural Alternative to Anti-Anxiety drugs and sleeping pills.* Rochester, VT: Park Street Press, 1996.

Kinzler, E., et al. "Effect of a special kava extract in patients with anxiety-, tension-, and excitation states of non-psychotic genesis. Double blind study with placebos over 4 weeks." *Arzneimittelforschung.* 1991; 41 (6): 584-588.

Kirch, P.V. "Indigenous agriculture on Uvea (Western Polynesia)." *Economic Botany.* 32, no. 2 (1978): 157-181.

Klohs, M.W., et al. "Piper Methysticum Forst. The synthesis of dl-methysticin and dl-dihydromethysticin." *J. Organic Chemistry.* 1959(24): 1829-1830.

Klohs, M.W., et al. "A chemical and pharmacological investigation of Piper methysticum Forst." *Journal of Medicine, Pharmacology, Chemistry.* 1 (1959): 95-99.

Klohs, M.W. and Keller, F. "A review of the chemistry and pharmacology of the constituents of Piper meth. Forst." *J. of Medicine, Pharm. & Chem.* 1 (1963): 95-103.

Klohs, M.W. "Chemistry of kava. In Ethnopharmacologic Search for Psychoactive Drugs." ed. Efron, D.H., et al.

Leach, E. "The structure of symbolism: Kava ceremony in Tonga." In: *The Interpretation of Ritual.* ed. La Fontaine, J.S., London: Tavistock, 1972.

Lebot, V., Merlin, M. and Lindstrom, L. *Kava: the Pacific Elixir.* Rochester, VT: Healing Arts Press, 1997.

Lehmann, E., et al. "Efficacy of a special Kava extract (Piper Methysticum) in patients with states of anxiety, tension and excitedness of non-mental origin. A double-blind placebo-controlled study of four weeks treatment." *Phytomedicine.* 1996, 3(2): 113-9.

Lemert, E.M. "Forms and pathology of drinking in three Polynesian societies." *American Anthropologist.* 1967 (66): 361-374.

Lemert, E.M. "Secular use of kava in Tonga." *Q. J. Stud. on Alcohol*. 1967(28): 328-341.

Lester, R.H. "Kava drinking in Vitu Levu, Fiji." *Oceania*. 12 (1941): 97-124.

Lewin, L. "Sur le Piper methysticum (kawa)." *Archives de Medecine et de Pharmacie Navale (Paris)*. 1886, 46: 210-220.

Lindenberg, D. and Pitule-Schodel, H. "D, L-Kavain in comparison with oxazepam in anxiety disorders. A double-blind study of clinical effectiveness." *Forschr. Med*. 108 (1990): 49-50, 53-54.

Lindstrom, L. "Drunkenness and gender on Tanna, Vanuatu." In: *Drugs in Western Pacific societies: relations of substance*, ed. Lindstrom, L., Assn. for Social Anthropology in Oceania. Monograph no. I 1. Lanham, Md.: University Press of America, 1987.

Lindstrom, L. "Grog blong yumi: Alcohol and kava on Tanna (Vanuatu)." In: *Through a glass darkly. Beer and modernisation in Papua, New Guinea*. ed. Marshall, M. Boroko: Institute for Social and Economic Research (IASER), 1982.

Lindstrom, L. "Speech and kava on Tanna." In: *Vanuatu: Politics, economics and ritual in island Melanesia*. ed. Allen, M. Sydney: Academic Press, 1981.

Lindstrom, L. "Spitting on Tanna." *Oceania*. 50 (1980): 228-234.

Maccuddin, R.C. *Samoan medicinal plants*. Pago Pago: Office of Comprehensive Health Planning, Department of Medicinal Services, Government of American Samoa, 1974.

Malauulu, J., et al. "Kava: Legends, ceremony, how-to-make and serve it." *Faasamoa Pea*. 1, no. 2 (1974): 20-37.

Mangnall, K. "Listen, it's kava night." *Pacific Islands Monthly*. 60 (1990): 25.

Marrazzi, A.S. "Electropharmacological and behavioral actions of kava." In: *Ethnopharmacologic Search for Psychoactive Drugs*. ed. Efron, D.H., et al.

Marshall, M. "Research bibliography of alcohol and kava studies in Oceania." *Micronesica*. 1974(10): 299-306.

Mathews, J.B., et al. "Effects of the heavy usage of kava on physical health: Summary of a pilot survey in an aboriginal community." *Med. J. of Australia*. 148 (1988): 548-555.

Meyer, H.J. "Pharmacology of kava: In Ethnopharmacologic Search for Psychoactive Drugs." ed. Efron, D.H., et al.

Munte, T.F., et al. "Effects of oxazepam and an extract of kava roots (Piper meth) on event-related potentials in a word recognition task." *Neuropsychobiology.* 1993; 27(1): 46-53.

Murray, M. *The Healing Power of Herbs.* Prima, 1995.

Naidu, R. "Kava: Problem or panacea?" *Islands Business.* (February 1983): 34-35.

Newell, W.H. "The kava ceremony in Tonga." *J. Polynesian Soc.* 56 (1947): 364-417.

Nolting, E. and Koop, A. "Sur la racine de kava." *Monitor Scientifique.* 1874, 14: 920-3.

Norton, S.A. and Ruze, P. "Kava dermopathy." *J. Am. Acad. Dermatol.* 1994 Jul; 31(1): 89-97.

Ott, J. *Pharmacotheon, Ethneogenic drugs, their plant sources and history.* Kennewick, Wash.: Natural Products Co., 1993.

Pfeiffer, C. C., et al. "Effect of kava in normal subjects and patients." In: *Ethnopharmacologic Search for Psycho-active Drugs.* ed. Efron, D.H., et al.

Prescott, J. and McCall, G., eds. "Kava: use and abuse in Australia and the South Pacific." National Drug and Alcohol Research Centre, Sydney, University of NSW Monograph No. 5. 1989: 13 - 25.

Rasmussen, A.K., Scheline, R.R., Solhein, E. and Hansel, R.. "Metabolism of some kava pyrones in the rat." *Zenobiotica.* 9 (1979): 1-16.

Raymond, W.V.D. "Kava (Piper methysticum Forst.)." *Colonial Plants and Animal Products.* 2 (1951): 46-52.

Russell, P.N., et al. "The effect of kava on altering and speed of access of information from long-term memory." *Bull. Psychonomic Soc.* 1987, 25(4): 236-237.

Ruze, P. "Kava-induced dermopathy: A niacin deficiency." *Lancet.* 335 (1990): 1442-1445.

Schelosky, L., et al. "Kava and dopamine antagonism" [letter]. *J. Neurol. Neurosurg. Psychiatry.* 1995 May; 58(5): 639-40.

Scheuer, P. and Horigan, T.J. "A new carbonyl compound from Piper Methysticum Forst." *Nature.* 1959 (184): 979-980.

Schleiffer, H., ed. *Sacred Narcotic Plants of the Old World: An Anthology of Texts from Ancient Times to the Present.* Introduction by Richard Evans Schultes. Monticello, N.Y.: Lubrecht & Cramer, 1979.

Scholing, W.E. and Clausen, H.D. "On the effect of dl-kavain: Experience with neuronika." *Med. Klin.* 72 (1977): 1301-1306.

Schubet, K. "Chemistry and pharmacology of kawa-kawa (Piper methysticum)." *Journal of the Society of Chemical Industry.* 43, no. 38 (1924): 766B.

Schultes, R.E. and A. Hofmann. *Plants of the Gods.* Rochester, Vt.: Healing Arts Press, 1992.

Serpenti, L.M. "On the social significance of an intoxicant (kava in New Guinea)." *Tropical Man.* 2 (1969): 31-44.

Shulgin, A.T. "The narcotic pepper: the chemistry and pharmacology of Piper methysticum and related species." *Bull. Narcotics.* 1973(25): 59-74.

Siegel, R.K. "Herbal intoxication." *JAMA.* 1976(236): 473-476.

Singh, Y.N. "A review of the historical, sociological and scientific aspects of kava and its uses in the South Pacific." *Fiji Medical Journal.* 9 (1981): 61-64.

Singh, Y.N. "Effects of kava on neuromuscular transmission and muscle contractility." *Journal of Ethnopharmacology.* 7 (1983): 267-276.

Singh, Y.N. *Kava: a bibliography.* Pacific Information Centre, University of the South Pacific, Suva. 1986.

Singh, Y.N. "Kava: An overview." *J. of Ethnopharmacology.* 37, no. 1 (1992): 13-45.

Singh, Y.N. and Blumenthal, M. "Kava: An overview." *Special Review, HerbalGram.* 1997, No. 39: 34-56.

Smiles, S. "Kava, the alcohol alternative (and why it's stronger in Vanuatu)." *Islands Business.* 1987 (May): 32-33.

Smith, R.M. "Pipermethystine: a novel pyridone alkaloid from Piper methysticum." *Tetrahedron Letters.* 35 (1979): 437-439.

Smith, R.M. "Kava lactones in Piper methysticum from Fiji." *Phytochemistry.* 22 (1983): 1055-1056.

Smith, R.M., et al. "High-performance liquid chromatography of kava lactones from Piper methysticum." *Journal of Chromatography.* 283 (1984):303-308.

Stafford, P. *Psychedelics Encyclopedia.* Third Expanded Edition. Berkeley, Calif.: Ronin Publishing, 1992.

Steinmetz, E.E. "Piper methysticum (kava). Famous drug plant of the South Seas Islands."*Amsterdam.* 1960. 1-46.

Suss, R. and Lehmann, P. "Hematogenous contact eczema cause by phytogenic drugs exemplified by kava root extract." *Hautarzt.* 1996 Jun; 47(6): 459-61.

Taofinu'u, P. "The kava ceremony is a prophecy." *Faasamoa Pea.* I (1974): 41-66.

Titcomb, M. "Kava in Hawaii." *Journal of Polynesian Society.* 57 (1948): 105-171.

Tora, V. *Yaqona in Fiji In Pacific rituals: Living or dying.* ed. Alufurai, A. Suva, Fiji: Institute of Pacific Studies, University of the South Pacific, 1986.

Turner, J.W. "The water of life: Kava ritual and the logic of sacrifice." *Ethnology.* 25 (1986): 203-214.

Van Veen, A.G. "Isolation and constitution of the narcotic substance from kawa kawa (Piper methysticum)." *Receuil des travaux chimiques des Pays-Bas.* 58 (1939): 521-527.

Volz, H.P. "Kava kava extract WS1490 versus placebo in anxiety disorder—a randomized, placebo-controlled 25 week outpatient trial." *Pharmacopsyc.* 1997, 30: 1-5.

Warnecke, G. "Neurovegetative dystonia in the female climacteric. Studies on the clinical efficacy and tolerance of kava extract WS 1490." *Forschr. Med.* 109 (1991): 120-122.

Weiss, R.F. *Herbal Medicine.* Beaconsfield, England: Beaconsfield Publishers, LTD, 1988.

Whistler, W.A. "Herbal medicine in the kingdom of Tonga." *Journal of Ethnopharmacology.* 31, no. 3 (1991): 339-372.

Whistler, W.A. *Polynesian Herbal Medicine.* Lawai, Hawaii: National Tropical Botanical Garden, 1992.

Whistler, W.A. "Traditional and herbal medicine in the Cook Islands." *Journal of Ethnopharmacology.* 13, no. 3 (1985): 239-280.

Winkelmann, R.K., et al. "Cutaneous syndrome sproduced as side effects of triparanol therapy." *Arch. Dermatol.* 1963 (87): 372-377.

Winzheimer, E. "Beitrage zur kenntnis de Kawawurzel." *Archiv. der Pharmazie.* 1908, 246: 338-365.

Young, R.L., et al. "Analysis of kava pyrones in extracts of Piper methysticum." *Phytochemistry.* 5 (1966): 795-798.

Yuncker, T.G. *Piperaceae of Micronesia.* Honolulu, Hawaii: Bernice P. Bishop Museum, 1959.

ADDITIONAL HEALTH TITLES FROM HOHM PRESS

TEN ESSENTIAL FOODS
by Lalitha Thomas

Lalitha has done for food what she did with such wit and wisdom for herbs in her best-selling *10 Essential Herbs*. This new book presents 10 ordinary, but *essential* and great-tasting foods that can: • Strengthen a weakened immune system • Rebalance brain chemistry • Fight cancer and other degenerative diseases • Help you lose weight, simply and naturally.

Carrots, broccoli, almonds, grapefruit and six other miracle foods will enhance your health when used regularly and wisely. Lalitha gives in-depth nutritional information plus flamboyant and good-humored stories about these foods, based on her years of health and nutrition counseling. Each chapter contains easy and delicious recipes, tips for feeding kids and helpful hints for managing your food dollar. A bonus section supports the use of 10 Essential Snacks.

This book's focus is squarely on target: fruits, vegetables and whole grains—everything comes in the right natural proportions."—Charles Attwood, M.D., F.A.A.P.; author, *Dr. Attwood's Low-Fat Prescription for Kids* (Viking).

Paper, 324 pages, $16.95   ISBN: 0-934252-74-2

• • •

10 ESSENTIAL HERBS, REVISED EDITION
by Lalitha Thomas

Peppermint. . .Garlic. . .Ginger. . .Cayenne. . .Clove. . . and 5 other everyday herbs win the author's vote as the "Top 10" most versatile and effective herbal applications for hundreds of health and beauty needs. *Ten Essential Herbs* offers fascinating stories and easy, step-by-step direction for both beginners and seasoned herbalists. Learn how to use cayenne for headaches, how to make a facial scrub with ginger, how to calm motion sickness and other stomach distress with peppermint, how to make slippery-elm cough drops for sore-throat relief. Special sections in each chapter explain the application of these herbs with children and pets too. **Over 25,000 copies in print.**

Paper, 396 pages, $16.95   ISBN: 0-934252-48-3

TO ORDER, PLEASE SEE ACCOMPANYING ORDER FORM.

ADDITIONAL HEALTH TITLES FROM HOHM PRESS

ARE YOU GETTING IT 5 TIMES A DAY?
Fruits and Vegetables
by Sydney H. Crackower, M.D., Barry A. Bohn, M.D. and
Rodney Langlinais, Reg. Pharmacist

The evidence is irrefutable. Research from around the world, and from the
American Cancer Society and the National Cancer Institute in the U.S.
agree ... 5 servings of nature's disease fighters—raw fruits and vegetables—
would markedly reduce cancer...stroke...and heart disease, the leading killers
of our times. Fresh fruits and vegetables, as well as an intelligently pursued
regimen of antioxidants, live enzymes and high fiber are the nutritional
basics of good health. This concise and straightforward book will give you
all the background research and practical steps you need to start getting it
today!

Paper, 78 pages, $ 6.95, ISBN: 0-934252-35-1

• • •

■ *HERBS, NUTRITION AND HEALING ;* AUDIO CASSETTE
SERIES
by Dr. Humbart "Smokey" Santillo, N.D.

Santillo's most comprehensive seminar series. Topics covered in-depth
include: • the history of herbology • specific preparation of herbs for
tinctures, salves, concentrates, etc. • herbal dosages in both acute and chronic
illnesses • use of cleansing and transition diets • treating colds and flu...
and more.

4 cassettes, 330 minutes, $40.00, ISBN: 0-934252-22-X

• • •

■ *NATURE HEALS FROM WITHIN;* AUDIO CASSETTE SERIES
by Dr. Humbart "Smokey" Santillo, N.D.

How to take the next step in improving your life and health through nutrition.
Topics include: • The innate wisdom of the body. • The essential role of
elimination and detoxification • Improving digestion • How "transition
dieting" will take off the weight—for good! • The role of heredity, diet, and
prevention in health • How to overcome tiredness, improve your immune
system and live longer...and happier.

1 cassette, $8.95, ISBN: 0-934252-66-1

TO ORDER, PLEASE SEE ACCOMPANYING ORDER FORM.

ADDITIONAL HEALTH TITLES FROM HOHM PRESS

NATURAL HEALING WITH HERBS
by Humbart Santillo, N.D.
Foreword by Robert S. Mendelsohn, M.D.

Dr. Santillo's first book, and Hohm Press' long-standing bestseller, is a classic handbook on herbal and naturopathic treatment. Acclaimed as the most comprehensive work of its kind, *Natural Healing With Herbs* details (in layperson's terms) the properties and uses of 120 of the most common herbs and lists comprehensive therapies for more than 140 common ailments. All in alphabetical order for quick reference. Includes special sections on: • Diagnosis • How to make herbal remedies • The nature of health and disease • Diet and detoxification • Homeopathy. . .and more. **Over 175,000 copies in print.**

Paper, 408 pages, $16.95   ISBN: 0-934252-08-4

• • •

FOOD ENZYMES - THE MISSING LINK TO RADIANT HEALTH
by Humbart "Smokey" Santillo, N.D.

Immune system health is a subject of concern for everyone today. This book explains how the body's immune system, as well as every other human metabolic function, requires enzymes in order to work properly. Food enzyme supplementation is more essential today than ever before, since stress, unhealthy food and environmental pollutants readily deplete enzymes from the body. Dr. Santillo's breakthrough book presents the most current research in this field and encourages simple, straightforward steps for how to make enzyme supplementation a natural addition to a nutrition-conscious lifestyle. Special sections on: • Longevity and disease • The value of raw food and juicing • Detoxification • Prevention of allergies and candida • Sports and nutrition.
Over 200,000 copies in print.
Paper, 108 pages, U.S. $7.95, ISBN: 0-934252-40-8 (English)

Now available in Spanish language version.
Paper, 108 pages, U.S. $6.95, ISBN: 0-934252-49-1 (Spanish)

■ Audio version of Food Enzymes
2 cassette tapes, 150 minutes, U.S. $17.95, ISBN: 0-934252-29-7

TO ORDER, PLEASE SEE ACCOMPANYING ORDER FORM.

ADDITIONAL HEALTH TITLES FROM HOHM PRESS

INTUITIVE EATING: **EveryBody's Guild to Vibrant Health and Lifelong Vitality Through Food**
by Humbart "Smokey" Santillo, N.D.

The natural voice of the body has been drowned out by the shouts of addictions, over-consumption, and devitalized and preserved foods. Millions battle the scale daily, experimenting with diets and nutritional programs, only to find their victories short-lived at best, confusing and demoralizing at worst. *Intuitive Eating* offers an alternative — a tested method for: • strengthening the immune system • natural weight loss • increasing energy • making the transition from a degenerative diet to a regenerative diet • slowing the aging process.

Paper, 444 pages, $16.95   ISBN: 0-934252-27-0

• • •

YOUR BODY CAN TALK: How to Use Simple Muscle Testing to Learn What Your Body Knows and Needs
by Susan L. Levy, D.C. and Carol Lehr, M.A.

The World's Most Advanced Diagnostic Health Tool is at your fingertips... Your Own Body can "talk" to you, telling you what it knows and needs for health and well-being. A simple method of **energetic muscle testing** can help you to decode symptoms and become sensitive to early warnings of body dysfunction...on a daily basis—long before life-threatening illness can develop. **This book will teach you how to use energetic Muscle Testing to:** • Discover your food sensitivities • Determine effects of electromagnetic pollution in your home or workplace • Evaluate the strength of your heart, your kidneys, your liver...• Test your immune system functioning • Choose which treatment methods will best handle your condition. Special Chapters for Women cover issues of PMS and Menopause. Special Chapter for Men deals with stress and heart disease, impotence and prostate problems.

Paper, 390 pages, $19.95   ISBN: 0-934252-68-8

TO ORDER, PLEASE SEE ACCOMPANYING ORDER FORM.

ADDITIONAL HEALTH TITLES FROM HOHM PRESS

DHEA: THE ULTIMATE REJUVENATING HORMONE
by Hasnain Walji, Ph.D.

This is the first published book about the age-slowing hormone, DHEA, which is fast being acknowledged as a new "wonder substance." Many studies indicate DHEA's positive usage for athletes and others concerned with losing weight without reducing caloric intake (DHEA blocks a fat-producing enzyme), as an aid to both short and long-term memory loss, and in such conditions as diabetes, cancer, Chronic Fatigue Syndrome, heart disease and immune system deficiencies. Contains a comprehensive but user-friendly review of research and relevant nutritional information.

Paper, 144 pages, $9.95   ISBN: 0-934252-70-X

• • •

MELATONIN AND AGING SOURCEBOOK
by Dr. Roman Rozencwaig, M.D. and Dr. Hasnain Walji, Ph.D.

"This is the most comprehensive reference of melatonin yet published. It is an indispensable tool for those scientists, researchers, and physicians engaged in anti-aging therapeutics."—Dr. Ronald Klatz, President, American Academy of Anti-aging Medicine.

This book covers the latest research on the pineal control of aging, melatonin and sleep, melatonin and immunity, melatonin's role in cancer treatment, antioxidant qualities of melatonin, dosages, contraindications, quality control, and use with other drugs, melatonin application to heart disease, Alzheimer's, diabetes, stress, major depression, seasonal affective disorders, AIDS, SIDS, cataracts, autism...and many other conditions.

Cloth, 220 pages, $79.95   ISBN: 0-934252-76-9

TO ORDER, PLEASE SEE ACCOMPANYING ORDER FORM.

ADDITIONAL TITLES OF INTEREST FROM HOHM PRESS

■ *LIVE SEMINAR ON FOOD ENZYMES*; AUDIO CASSETTE SERIES
by Dr. Humbart "Smokey" Santillo, N.D.

An in-depth discussion of the properties of food enzymes, describing their valuable use to maintain vitality, immunity, health and longevity. A must for anyone interested in optimal health. Complements all the information in the book.

1 cassette, $8.95, ISBN: 0-934252-29-7

• • •

■ *FRUITS AND VEGETABLES—The Basis of Health*; AUDIO CASSETTE SERIES
by Dr. Humbart "Smokey" Santillo, N.D.

Juicing of fruits and vegetables is one of the fastest and most efficient ways to supply the body with the raw food nutrients and enzymes needed to maintain optimal health. Explains the essential difference between a live food diet, which heals the body, and degenerative foods, which weaken the immune system and cause disease. Recipes included.

1 cassette, $8.95, ISBN: 0-934252-65-3

• • •

■ *WEIGHT-LOSS SEMINAR*; AUDIO CASSETTE SERIES
by Dr. Humbart "Smokey" Santillo, N.D.

"The healthiest people in the world know the secret of weight loss," says Santillo in this candid, practical, and information-based seminar. "If your body is getting what it needs, the appetite automatically turns off!" The reason for overweight is that we are starving ourselves to death, based on the improper balance of nutrients from our current food sources. This seminar explains the worthlessness of most dietary regimens and explodes many common myths about weight gain. Santillo stresses: • The essential distinction between "good" fats and "bad" fats • The necessity for protein and how to use it efficiently • How to get our primary vitamins and minerals from food • How to ease into becoming an "intuitive eater" so that the body is always getting what it knows it needs.

1 cassette, $8.95, ISBN: 0-934252-75-0

ADDITIONAL HEALTH TITLES FROM HOHM PRESS

KAVA: Nature's Relaxant For Anxiety, Stress and Pain
by Hasnain Walji, Ph.D.

KAVA is currently one of the hottest products in the natural medicine and health-food trade. This book provides consumers with a readable introduction and a balanced and authoritative treatment of this timely subject. Today, a growing body of scientific research is corroborating the experience of age-old folk medicine, that KAVA does indeed possess healing, analgesic and anesthetic qualities. KAVA has been shown to relieve the anxiety, tension and restlessness that characterize STRESS, a major contributing factor in the most deadly diseases of our times. Hasnain Walji, Ph.D. is a researcher, writer and freelance journalist specializing in holistic health, nutrition and complementary therapies. He is a prolific author with over 20 books to his credit, including *Melatonin* (Harper-Collins, 1995) and *DHEA: The Ultimate Rejuvenating Hormone* (Hohm Press, 1996).

Paper, 144 pages, $9.95   ISBN: 0-934252-78-5

RETAIL ORDER FORM FOR HOHM PRESS HEALTH BOOKS

Name_____ Phone (   ) _____

Street Address or P.O. Box _____

City _____State _____ Zip Code _____

	QTY	TITLE	ITEM PRICE	TOTAL PRICE	
1		10 ESSENTIAL FOODS	$16.95		
2		10 ESSENTIAL HERBS	$16.95		
3		ARE YOU GETTING IT 5 TIMES A DAY?	$6.95		
4		DHEA: The Ultimate Rejuvenating Hormone	$9.95		
5		FOOD ENZYMES/ENGLISH	$7.95		
6		FOOD ENZYMES/SPANISH	$6.95		
7		FOOD ENZYMES BOOK/AUDIO	$17.95		
8		FRUITS & VEGETABLES/AUDIO	$8.95		
9		HERBS, NUTRITION AND HEALING/AUDIO	$40.00		
10		INTUITIVE EATING	$16.95		
11		LIVE SEMINAR ON FOOD ENZYMES/AUDIO	$8.95		
12		THE MELATONIN AND AGING SOURCEBOOK	$79.95		
13		NATURAL HEALING WITH HERBS	$16.95		
14		NATURE HEALS FROM WITHIN/AUDIO	$8.95		
15		WEIGHT LOSS SEMINAR/AUDIO	$8.95		
16		YOUR BODY CAN TALK: How to Use...	$19.95		
17		KAVA: Nature's Relaxant...	$9.95		

SURFACE SHIPPING CHARGES

1st book $4.00
Each additional item $1.00

SUBTOTAL:	
SHIPPING: (see below)	
TOTAL:	

SHIP MY ORDER

☐ Surface U.S. Mail—Priority   ☐ UPS (Mail + $2.00)
☐ 2nd-Day Air (Mail + $5.00)   ☐ Next-Day Air (Mail + $15.00)

METHOD OF PAYMENT:

☐ Check or M.O.   Payable to Hohm Press, P.O. Box 2501, Prescott, AZ 86302
☐ Call 1-800-381-2700 to place your credit card order
☐ Or call 1-520-717-1779 to fax your credit card order
☐ Information for Visa/MasterCard order only:

Card #_____–_____–_____–_____ Expiration Date _____

ORDER NOW! Call 1-800-381-2700 or fax your order to 1-520-717-1779.
(Remember to include your credit card information.)